Martin Lawrence and Peter Pritchard (Eds.)

GENERAL PRACTITIONER EDUCATION

UK and Nordic Perspectives

Springer-Verlag
London Berlin Heidelberg New York
Paris Tokyo Hong Kong
Barcelona Budapest

Martin Lawrence, MRCP FRCGP
Senior Lecturer in General Practice,
University of Oxford, Fellow of Green College,
Rapporteur UK-Nordic Workshop,
Department of Public Health and Primary Care,
Gibson Building, Radcliffe Infirmary,
Oxford OX2 6HE, UK

Peter Pritchard, MA FRCGP
Senior Medical Adviser,
Advanced Computation Laboratory,
Imperial Cancer Research Fund,
Coordinator of UK-Nordic Workshop,
31 Martin's Lane, Dorchester on Thames,
Wallingford, Oxford OX10 8JF, UK

ISBN-13:978-3-540-19741-6 e-ISBN-13:978-1-4471-1960-9
DOI: 10.1007/978-1-4471-1960-9

British Library Cataloguing in Publication Data
Lawrence, Martin, *1943–*
General practitioner education: UK and Nordic perspectives
I. Title II. Pritchard, Peter
610.71141
ISBN-13:978-3-540-19741-6

Library of Congress Data Available

2112/3830-543210 Printed on acid-free paper

PREFACE

Vocational training and continuing education are in a state of rapid change and development in Nordic countries; in the United Kingdom there is a serious upheaval and reappraisal as a result of the review of the National Health Service. In the past, the UK has been seen as a pioneer and as a model for vocational training. Now, several Nordic countries are making very rapid progress and innovating methods of small group learning, both for vocational training and continuing medical education (CME).

A workshop to look at strategies, methods of implementation and evaluation of vocational training and CME was held in June 1990 in London. The aim was to learn from each other's ideas and experience. The topics were chosen after an extensive questionnaire study of leading general practitioners in Nordic countries and UK.

This publication includes papers written by contributors to the workshop, and also the pre-circulated papers which described the health systems and educational realities in the six countries: Denmark, Finland, Iceland, Norway, Sweden and UK.

Evaluation of the workshop itself was very positive, and it was seen as a landmark in development of general practitioner education which has implications for many countries outside Northern Europe.

November 1991 — Peter Pritchard

INTRODUCTION

The benefits to be derived from a UK-Nordic workshop on vocational and continuing education arise from the political, structural and sociological similarities between the countries. They are similar enough to be relevant to each other, but different enough each to offer possible benefits to the others.

The similarities are striking. We all have registered lists and so have personal responsibility; the service is free or heavily subsidized; and population coverage is comprehensive.

On the other hand some of us are self-employed, some salaried. We have different contracts which result in different working conditions and primary care team structures, and we use different educational systems. (The main characteristics for each country have been summarized in the descriptive papers – section 7).

So what did we learn? Perhaps first, the British GPs learned that the word for teaching and learning in Norwegian, Danish and Swedish is the same, *uddannelse*. We need to remember that teaching cannot be considered except in the context of learning.

Most importantly, we learned that practice depends on circumstances – the structure of the service, time, money, geography; and that education depends on practice. So for example, systems are well developed – to the point perhaps of being rigid – in the UK, where there have been good funds, group practices and the central development of standards. In Norway and Denmark practitioners are much more isolated, either by geography or single-handedness; education tends to be in groups and there is less emphasis on management and preventive care and more on relationships. In Sweden and Finland doctors are salaried and responsible for a geographic area; there is a lack of doctors but a well developed team approach to caring for the community.

Each country has developed systems to respond to its own particular circumstances – postgraduate groups in sparsely populated Norway; in-practice education for the primary health care teams of the UK; 12 man groups for the single-handed GPs of Denmark; re-accreditation projects for the re-emerging general practitioners of Sweden; and a strong university component from Finland. But there are also the commonalities: the need for self-direction, the imperative of teaching teachers, and the move to continuing formative assessment.

Above all we learned to reconsider our values. All the countries teach on the basis of knowledge, skills and attitudes; we began to believe that values have a more positive significance than attitudes. Our views on knowledge and skills diverge little, but the way in which we esteem different parts of our learning or practice vary hugely, and are a critical area for debate. For instance, the UK seems well 'ahead' in many areas of teaching and assessment; but do UK teachers really teach and assess the areas of general practice that are the most important, or are some of the Scandinavian approaches, with less structure but more appreciation of the individual, more valid? The answer surely lies in a synthesis of the two approaches.

The first part of this book reviews teaching under five headings, each introduced by a brief commentary highlighting the main issues and indicating the consensus view. The second part consists of papers, produced prior to the workshop; comparing the structure of health care systems and general practice education in the UK and Nordic countries.

November 1991 Martin Lawrence

Acknowledgements

The editors wish to thank all those who supported the UK-Nordic Workshop 1990, in particular Hässle Läkemedel AB, the Medical Insurance Agency, the British United Provident Association, the Department of Health, Parke-Davis Research Laboratories, the International Committee of the Royal College of General Practitioners and Merck Sharp and Dohme Ltd.

The UK-Nordic Medical Educational Trust has helped with the cost of publication. Sue Flanders and Lisbet Clements processed the text.

CONTENTS

CONTRIBUTORS

Dr Jamie Bahrami United Kingdom
Regional Adviser in General Practice, Yorkshire. Senior Lecturer in General Practice, Leeds University. Course Organiser for Vocational Training Scheme. Examiner, Royal College of General Practitioners. Founder of the National Association of Course Organisers (UK).

Dr Niels Bentzen Denmark
Senior Lecturer in General Practice, Department of Community Health, University of Odense.

Dr Per Blicher-Hansen Denmark
General Practitioner. Leader of Theoretical Vocational Training, Copenhagen. Head of the Committee on Vocational Training in Denmark.

Dr Graham Buckley United Kingdom
General Practitioner, Livingston, near Edinburgh. Associate Adviser in General Practice, South East Scotland. Lately, Editor, British Journal of General Practice (formerly Journal of the Royal College of General Practitioners).

Dr Nicolaj Friderichsen Denmark
General Practitioner and Teacher, Ærösköbing.

Dr Anna-Karin Furhoff Sweden
General Practitioner and Lecturer, Institute of General Practice, Karolinska Institute, Stockholm. Formerly Head of Division of Primary Health Care, National Board of Health and Welfare, Stockholm. Responsible for training of future general practitioners (1980 – 1987), and for continuing education in a Stockholm district.

Professor Denis Pereira Gray United Kingdom
Professor of General Practice, Exeter University Institute of Postgraduate Medicine. Regional Adviser in General Practice, University of Bristol. Honorary Editor of College Publications, Royal College of General Practitioners. Chairman of Council, Royal College of General Practitioners. Formerly Editor, Journal of the Royal College of General Practitioners.

Dr John Hasler United Kingdom
Regional Postgraduate Adviser in General Practice. Former Honorary Secretary and Chairman of Council, Royal College of General Practitioners. Author/editor of several books and research papers.

Dr John Horder United Kingdom
Visiting Professor, Royal Free Hospital Medical School, London. Past President, Royal College of General Practitioners. Past Consultant and Travelling Fellow, World Health Organization. Co-author, 'The Future General Practitioner: learning and teaching', and of numerous other publications on education.

Bjørn Hoftvedt Norway
Director, Educational Unit, Norwegian Medical Association.

Dr Donald Irvine United Kingdom
Northern Regional Adviser in General Practice. Chairman, Joint Committee of Postgraduate Training for General Practice. Chairman, Standards Committee of General Medical Council. Former Honorary Secretary and Chairman of Council, Royal College of General Practitioners. Co-author, 'The Future General Practitioner: learning and teaching'.

Professor Mauri Isokoski Finland
Professor of General Practice, University of Tampere.

Dr Mogens Johansen Denmark
General Practitioner and Medical Examiner, Vejle. Consultant, Danish Medical Association. Regional coordinator of continuing medical education.

Dr Sirkka Keinänen-Kiukaanniemi Finland
Associate Professor in General Practice, University of Oulu. Assistant Chairman of the Association of General Practitioners of Finland since 1989. Author of papers connected with research topics.

Dr Claes Kjær Denmark
Lecturer in General Practice, University of Copenhagen. Director of Postgraduate Education.

Professor James Knox United Kingdom
Professor of General Practice, University of Dundee.

Dr Katia Käyhkö Finland
Senior Lecturer in General Practice, University of Helsinki.

Dr Martin Lawrence United Kingdom
Senior Lecturer in General Practice, University of Oxford. Fellow of Green College. Rapporteur, UK-Nordic Workshop.

Professor John Maeland Norway
Associate Professor, Institute of General Practice, University of Bergen.

Dr Marshall Marinker United Kingdom
Director, MSD Foundation, London. Formerly Professor of General Practice, University of Leicester. Chairman of Education Division, Royal College of General Practitioners. Co-author, 'The Future General Practitioner: learning and teaching'.

Dr Bengt Mattsson Sweden
Clinical Reader in General Practice, University of Umeå.

Professor David Metcalfe United Kingdom
Professor of General Practice, University of Manchester. Author of numerous papers on teaching and on research interests.

Dr Marjukka Mäkelä Finland
Senior Lecturer in General Practice, University of Helsinki.

Dr Christina Nerbrand Sweden
Vice President, Swedish Association of General Practitioners.

Dr Peter Pritchard United Kingdom
Senior Medical Adviser, Advanced Computation Laboratory, Imperial Cancer Research Fund. Coordinator, UK-Nordic Workshop.

Professor Jóhann Sigurdsson Iceland
Professor of General Practice, University of Reykjavik.

Dr Jørund Straand Norway
Lecturer, Institute of General Practice, University of Bergen, Norway.

Dr Wenche Telstad Norway
General Practitioner, Mehamm. Vice President, Norwegian Medical Association.

Dr Margareta Troein Sweden
General Practitioner. Department of Community Health Sciences, University of Lund. Chairman, standing committee on GP vocational training, National Board of Health.

Dr Irma Virjo Finland
Senior Lecturer in Primary Health Care, University of Tampere.

Professor Steinar Westin Norway
Professor of General Practice and Community Medicine, University of Trondheim. Author, 'Research in General Practice' (1983), 'An Educational Handbook for General Practitioners' (1985) and 'Problem Solving and Decision Making in General Practice' (1987) and papers on research interests.

1. STRATEGIES FOR VOCATIONAL TRAINING

Discussion points

'The secret of general practice is to hold
self-contradictory concepts with confidence'.
E G Buckley

The varying methods and directions of vocational training exemplify the truth of this statement, a truth emphasized by the similarities and differences between UK and Nordic countries. There must be a multi-faceted programme of education in knowledge, skills and the development of values, yet there remains the necessity of training; we agree on the desirability of self-directed learning yet the need for a core curriculum; and on the values of academic freedom but the demand for accreditation. The issues are well illustrated in comparing the highly developed UK programmes with the systems of vocational training in Scandinavia which are less well supervised but perhaps more effective at addressing doctors' and patients' values.

Delegates were universally concerned that problem-oriented teaching and self-directed learning should permeate the programmes more widely, especially to indicate awareness of the need of lifelong education. There was agreement that the GP's role must be defined so that aims can be developed before any teaching programme is designed; and that any teaching programme should involve the hospital phase of vocational training, not just the part in practice. The Danes aim to put the practice part of vocational training early, so that later hospital training relates to it. The Norwegians have attained 40 out of 56 weeks in practice, but the learning is largely unsupervised (Figure 1.1).

The need for teaching teachers was fully accepted, but only widely undertaken in the United Kingdom and Norway. Its effectiveness depends on time and incentives - these were fully available in the UK when the scheme got under way in the early 1970s. It is doubtful that such funding would have been available today, and other countries are faced with the problem of acquiring funds.

Along with finance and incentives go the possibilities of teacher training and selection. Currently, incentives for training in the United Kingdom are high and the issues of quality have been emphasised: in Nordic countries the incentives are smaller, so pressures which can be exerted on trainers are less also. This results in less training of teachers and a lower threshold for selection of practices. The looser systems in Scandinavia give their teachers concern over the standard of training especially in terms of quality assurance, but enable great freedom to develop young doctors' values: worries in the UK centre more over the need to retain the important values in a centrally directed system. There is great opportunity to learn as we move towards each other.

STRATEGIES FOR VOCATIONAL TRAINING

Graham Buckley - United Kingdom

Big questions lead to uncertain answers. What is the appropriate strategy for the vocational training of future general practitioners? This is certainly a big question and has led me to read authors as varied as Karl Popper, Arthur Koestler, Jacob Bronowski and Marshall Marinker. Apart from sharing a middle European ancestry, what do a philosopher, an author, a scientist and a doctor have in common? One shared characteristic has been their unconventional and innovative approach to definitions within science and the educational opportunities offered at boundaries between disciplines.

Definitions

The traditional conventional starting point for defining strategies is to seek to establish what we are trying to achieve. In vocational training we are trying to develop good general practitioners. This is a self-evident and virtually useless statement. What is a good general practitioner? What is general practice? Previous attempts to define general practice, for example by the Leeuwenhorst Group and, more recently, WONCA, do not excite the blood. Even less exciting are the detailed descriptions of the content of general practice as outlined in the 'Future General Practitioner' and in the Netherlands Curriculum.

If we over-emphasize content in our strategies for vocational training, we may repeat the mistakes of undergraduate education. Styles in his recent Pickles Lecture describes phenomena such as 'curriculosclerosis' or 'hardening of the categories', 'curriculomegaly' and even cancer of the curriculum. The possible distorting effect on education of a rigidly defined curriculum needs to be taken seriously. A continuing controversy in the United Kingdom is the way in which the Membership examination for The Royal College of General Practitioners imposes a curriculum upon vocational training.

Hidden Curriculum

Rather than concentrating on content, I wish to emphasise the value and influence of the hidden curriculum. Marinker has eloquently pointed out that we remember who taught us, not what was taught. Oscar Wilde may not be a good role model but he did say 'The most important things in life cannot be taught'. However, we can provide the context in which the important things in general practice can be learned. My personal view of the ideal qualities of a general practitioner is that he or she should show: care, compassion, warmth, flexibility, stamina and wit. I submit that these are characteristics, not a definition of the ideal general practitioner. The process of developing or acquiring these qualities is a social one akin to growing up in a family. It is therefore a type of maturation process.

Hospital training seen in this light can be seen to be similar to a neglectful and abusive family in which unrealistic demands are made on the individual. Problems are denied, there is indirect communication with authority figures and the junior feels to be isolated and unheard.

Social Aspects of Vocational Training

The social elements within vocational training tend to be viewed as optional enjoyable extras. I think this is a wrong concept. Social elements are central and crucial in the development of future general practitioners. One of the main tasks of the tutor is to provide a stimulating and supportive environment in which the educational expectations and demands are individually tailored to the needs of the young doctor.

At the end of vocational training, we wish doctors to be enthusiastic and confident, yet self-critical and open to external criticism. For their future careers, the young doctors should know how to seek and receive help. There is a paradox at the heart of clinical medicine. In order to be effective doctors, they need to be confident in the way in which they interact with patients, yet in order for medicine to progress, doctors need to retain their scientific scepticism and their awareness that there is much uncertainty in clinical practice.

Do training practices and trainers have the ability to help young doctors in this maturational process? The practical resources within a practice may reflect these abilities, but not necessarily. The importance of the personal relationship between trainer and trainee is most evident when it goes wrong. The powerful emotional reactions show that there is more involved in the educational process than the simple transfer of information from an experienced to an inexperienced doctor.

Characteristics of Vocational Training Release Courses

We start our release course with a short residential course in a comfortable country hotel. The content of the three day course is demanding. This introduction shows that the tutors value the young doctors but also have high expectations of them.

The release course itself is generally referred to as 'playschool'. I take this to be a compliment in that it shows that the experience is generally an enjoyable one. The basis of it.is small group discussion in which within a group of peers there is gradual exposure of the individual within a protected and supportive environment in which feelings of uncertainty and inadequacy can be shared.

In the current educational jargon, assessment of the trainees during their training year is formative. Individual trainees can see how they perform in comparison to their colleagues. The assessment feedback is confidential to the individual concerned. The assessment techniques cover multiple choice questions, patient management questions, performance in OSCE and responses to questionnaires about coping and confidence. The assessment is popular in the early months of the trainee year but less so as the doctors reach the end of their general practice year.

Projects

Project work is given particular emphasis within my group of 10 trainees. There are no rules about the content of the project. Trainees are simply asked to look at one aspect of general practice and report their findings back to the group. Most choose to examine aspects of their own training practice but the project could be a literature review. My reason in encouraging trainees to do this work is that it is a creative and individual approach to adult learning in which the trainee's own ideas are formulated and submitted to a peer group for comment. It is akin to the way in which further education takes place in the humanities. It emphasises that vocational training is education as well as training.

Bronowski writing about science and human values identifies three essential qualities in science: creativity, habit of truth, and a sense of human dignity. This leads me to conjecture on how vocational training should prepare young doctors for their future role in society.

Future Role of Doctors

James McCormack has described general practitioners as father figures and plumbers. In the past, general practitioners were also leaders within communities. We need to take on this role again. In order to fulfil this, we need to be educated and not just trained. We need a breadth of understanding about the tide of history and the cultural context in which our patients live. We need to embrace a wider role as well as our one-to- one contact with patients.

Strategies for Creativity

If doctors are to take on leadership roles within the community, and if vocational training is to grow and develop, then the most important strategy is one which encourages creativity. It is important not only for the future of the individual doctor but also for our discipline. Without new insights and fresh approaches, there is the danger that general practice will become mechanistic and repetitive. Audit and protocols may drive us in this direction. Uncertainty lies at the heart not only of general practice but also at the heart of science. Physicists are now having to deal with the mathematics of chaos. In behavioural science, uncertainty is even more obvious. I find this inevitable uncertainty a liberating concept which provides the opportunity for all doctors to be involved in research. We should encourage our trainees to question.

Boundaries and Conclusion

I started this lecture by citing influential thinkers who have been concerned with boundaries. Tillich has also looked at phenomena of boundaries. He notes that the boundary is the best place for acquiring knowledge but at the cost of peace of mind. In general practice there is the boundary between individual and population medicine, health and illness, physical and psychological disorders, art and science, trainee and principal. Indeed general practice, rather than an entity, can be thought of as one continuous boundary.

STRATEGIES FOR VOCATIONAL TRAINING

Per Blicher-Hansen - Denmark

Strategies can be considered under headings: WHAT? - WHO? -WHERE? - WHEN? and HOW? The big question WHAT? will be divided up into three parts - knowledge, skills and attitudes.

Knowledge. Categories of knowledge include the following:

Diseases and their handling in the particular context of the doctor in general practice.

Prevention, related to specific diseases, social groups or surroundings. This also includes the knowledge of preventive work of other groups, eg nurses.

Family life. The dynamics in the family, the problems of generations and the problems of loneliness.

The influence of social and local surroundings upon the individuals and the response of the individual to that influence.

Problem solving methods at hand for the general practitioner.

Rules of conduct specific to our profession. For example: patient-doctor, doctor-doctor, doctor-authority and doctor-social worker relationships.

Research methods applicable to general practice.

Legislation of social medicine and its influence on the patient.

Skills - specific for general practice in contrast to hospital work

The use of communication, diagnostic procedures and treatment.

The identification and correct management of risk groups by screening procedures and preventive medicine.

The use of epidemiological knowledge in general practice.

Proper decision making concerning the problems presented - together with the patients, the family and the authorities.

Awareness of time, and its use as a therapeutical and organizational aid.

Cooperation with all categories of staff, professional or non-medical groups.

Clinic organization, including economics, staff training and cooperation, research and teaching

Attitudes

The ability to identify with the situation and to establish a personal and effective cooperation with the patient,

The ability to bring forward the natural resources of the patient,

Willingness to evaluate both the positive and negative sides of your own work,

The realisation of the need for continuing education. This is of very great importance and that is one of the things we are going to strengthen in Denmark.

These items: knowledge, skills and attitudes are the 'WHAT?s' that vocational training must include. I think that we can agree on this, but the ways of implementation are different in each country.

In Denmark, as of course in other countries, we feel a great need for improvement and we are trying hard to intensify research in primary health care, which is the only way of improving our service and teaching. We have research units at the Copenhagen University and very soon coming at the University of Aarhus. We have two research tutors outside the University to help and to encourage general practitioners in this specific field.

The need for systems and collection of data implies that computers will be used on a much broader scale. The establishment of sentinel practices is just around the corner and this will definitely contribute to a much better description of our profession.

Medical audit has got off to a very slow start in Denmark, but for the past two years it has been intensified. Recently a medical audit handbook has been produced and sent out to all general practitioners in Denmark. So, I find it very necessary to emphasize the need for research in order to improve vocational training.

WHO? Who is going to communicate what aspect of the profession to the trainees?

In all our countries we have clinical and theoretical training. In the training general practitioners participate, and so do specialists, social workers and many others. Unfortunately in Denmark it is only during the 12 months in general practice and at the compulsory theoretical course, that general practitioners are in charge of the education. We are at this moment working on a project, in which we try to extend the education given at the theoretical course on to the years when the trainees are still at hospitals before establishing their own general practices. As there may elapse several years from the end of the theoretical course before having your own practice in Denmark, we find it very important to maintain the mind of the trainees in the way of thinking of general practice.

This is to emphasize that we must intensify the elements of vocational training which take place in general practice. It is not possible to have an education for primary health care which is mainly taught by specialists in other fields.

WHERE? Where are the trainees to be made familiar with the various aspects of the profession?

This seems to be a very simple question, but nevertheless there is great variety in where the vocational training is actually taking place.

Let us compare Denmark and Norway. In Denmark only six months out of 42 take place in general practice, whereas in Norway four years out of five are in general practice - with an advanced tutorial function to support the training. To this you can add the basic clinical training of 18 months which is similar in the two countries, where six months are in general practice, (see figure 1.1).

WHEN? When is a particular aspect introduced? What should come first and what comes later?

Again there is a great variety among the countries present here and that of course depends on the structural differences already mentioned. Will we be able to systematise the structure of the vocational training and so set up a scheme dealing with this question? If not the management of WHEN? will not be in the near future.

HOW? How is an aspect of professional work best introduced?

How do we create the best conditions for training the future general practitioners? How do we train the trainers? How do we assess, if the objectives have been achieved?

The future of vocational training

If I were to describe the ideal of vocational training it would be like this:

Beginning at the university with compulsory education in general practice. This seems to be so obvious, but nevertheless it's only a few years ago that general practice became compulsory and a subject in the final examination in Denmark.

In the basic clinical training for all doctors it is essential that six months takes place in primary health care. This has been the intention in Denmark since 1974 but it will not become reality until 1991! It is of great importance to the cooperation between primary health care and the hospitals, that all doctors have seen and know the working conditions of general practice, especially in our country where the general practitioner is the first person to take care of the patient.

When the young doctor has decided to enter vocational training for general practice the theoretical course should be rather early, eg one year after the basic clinical training.

It is important to follow the trainee during his or her work at the hospitals after the theoretical course. There must be return days and tutorial groups to keep the trainee in the habit of thinking of primary health care - and not to submit to the hospital way of thinking. Consequently groups of 10-14 persons have experimented with frequent meetings, discussions and evaluation of their working methods and knowledge, and as such are the perfect basis for continuing education for the rest of their working lives. In this schedule there is a continuous line of education going on from the student years through vocational training to continuing education.

In 1992 there will be free interchange of manpower in the European Community, which will also facilitate the coordination of medical education inside the EEC. Only Denmark of the Scandinavian countries is in the EEC, but in Denmark we feel a great need to have equivalent education in all the Scandinavian countries, which for the moment is not the case. General practitioners in Denmark are not regarded as specialists. This implies that we are not allowed to work freely as general practitioners in other Scandinavian countries even though we are so much alike, and even though we seldom have any language problems.

Inside the EEC all member countries in 1987 subscribed to a directive under the Treaty of Rome, which required them to start to establish training courses for intending general practitioners in 1988. By 1995 all general practitioners wishing to work in the social security systems of the member countries will need to have been trained. The standard required is a two year period of full-time postgraduate training of which at least six months are spent in an approved practice.

Until recently Denmark seemed to be the leader of vocational training, but as pointed out before we have now 42 months of vocational training and only six months in general practice. That means that we nearly have gone to the minimum requirements inside the EEC.

Looking to the future I hope to see general practitioners from the United Kingdom and the Scandinavian countries all having an equivalent amount of vocational training. As our socio-economical development seems to be so much alike, we shall gain in professional strength and in the efficiency of our continuing education, provided that we can harmonize our vocational training. If Denmark can be a leader of vocational training, this could be an example for the rest of Europe.

Finally, in order to explain why I have spoken so much about Denmark and our own conditions, I will quote Piet Hein - a famous Danish scientist, writer, poet and inventor. He said that smallness should not be underrated, and:

> 'Denmark seen from foreign land
> looks but like a grain of sand.
> Denmark as we Danes conceive it
> is so big you won't believe it'.

Fig 1.1

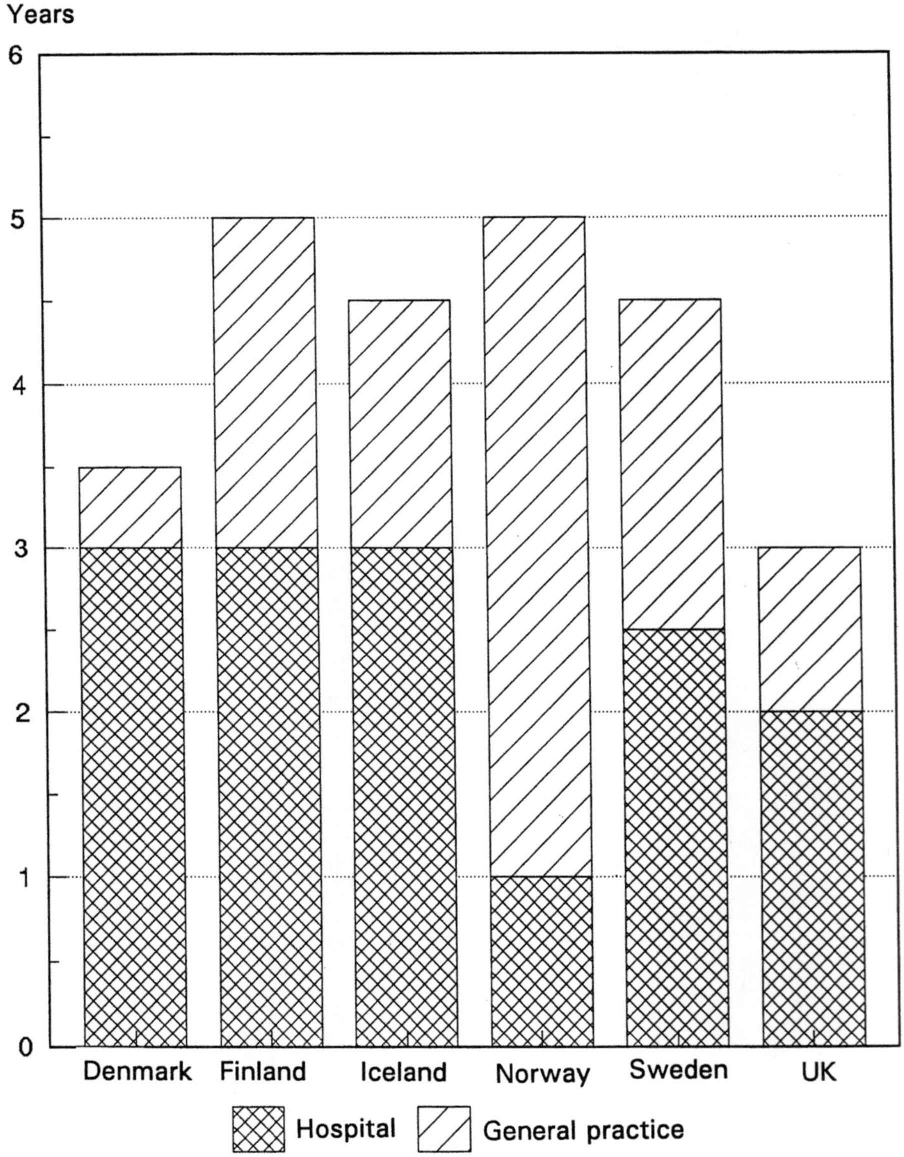

Vocational training for general practice indicating period of service in general practice and at hospital.

2. STRATEGIES FOR CONTINUING EDUCATION

Discussion points

> 'Compulsory continuing education with re-certification could be regarded as the failure of a profession to convince society that it is capable of maintaining standards itself'.
>
> Anna-Karin Furhoff

The struggle to know how to design continuing medical education is common to all the UK-Nordic countries. In such a large field as general practice the struggle is to know what is important, and how to motivate all doctors to participate.

Self-directed learning appears crucial: this form of teaching and learning should begin at medical school, permeate pre-registration teaching and progress through vocational training, in order to emphasise the continuing need for CME throughout life. A major problem here is that funding, except in Sweden, is different for each section, varying between the university (undergraduate), health services (vocational training), and self-provided (continuing education).

Thereafter repeated peer review and assessment should determine each doctor's programme of continuing education. This can take many forms - 'What sort of Doctor?' or 'Fellowship by Assessment' in the UK; re-accreditation based groups in Norway; 12 man groups in Denmark for example. It was generally agreed that education programmes based on groups concentrating on performance review are the way forward.

The structure and motivation is different and variable. In Scandinavia, where GPs are usually salaried or single-handed, groups outside practice are popular: in the UK where group practice is the norm the practice team often forms an educational group. There needs to be a balance between in-practice and external education, just as there needs to be a balance between the content of learning determined by quality assurance and the flexibility of self-directed learning addressing each doctor's needs and values.

Motivation and provision vary widely. For instance, Icelandic GPs have 15 days paid per year; in Denmark there is little compulsion and no financial support; the UK has the postgraduate education allowance (PGEA) which is conditional on attendance; Sweden relies heavily on industry support; and in Finland most courses are provided by the university. Time is money and the success of CME will depend on both, as well as on doctors' motivation.

STRATEGIES FOR CONTINUING EDUCATION

Anna-Karin Furhoff - Sweden

The ethical imperative and society's needs

The words profession and occupation are both translated by the Swedish word "yrke". It might be profitable to explore why two words are necessary in English, when one is enough in Swedish. Here are some quotations that could help us to understand what is special about a profession.

> A profession is "a vocation whose practice is founded upon an understanding of a theoretical structure of some department of learning or science".
>
> M.L.Cogan, 1953

> "Professionals profess. They profess to know better than others the nature of certain matters, and to know better than their clients what ails them or their affairs. This is the essence of the professional idea and the professional claim. From it flow many consequences...."
>
> E.Hughes, 1963

One consequence is that the code of ethics of any profession - and a code of ethics is a characteristic of a profession - contains a commitment to life-long learning. That is the only way in which a profession can guarantee its clients that its practitioners really know best and are worthy of the confidence placed in them.

Usually, well-functioning professions are regarded as valuable to society and are protected by legislation. The organization which issues the licence to practise guarantees both that new practitioners are competent, and also that they shall remain so in the future by supervising professional practice. Naturally, society demands something in return for this protection. The privileges of the medical profession, for example, can only be extended to those who remain masters of their branch of learning throughout their professional lives.

Thus, to the ethical imperative of continuing education, we may add a demand from the public. If professionals neglect the constant renewing of their knowledge and skills, society will take measures. In this context, a compulsory continuing education with re-certification could be regarded as the failure of a profession to convince society that it is capable of meeting these demands itself.

Characteristics of CME

The basis of continuing medical education (CME) is that knowledge is impermanent. The world we live in also changes, and with it the needs of our patients. The knowledge, skills and insights that CME is to provide then depend not only on what new knowledge has become available, but also on the specific needs of the doctor.

Only the doctors themselves can analyse their needs - a process requiring not only insight into previous knowledge but also into their practice, that is to say, the needs of their patients. Consequently, each doctor must play an active part in planning of his or her CME.

Most importantly, CME depends on the motivation of the doctor. Only strong motivation, whether founded on professional ethics or fear of reprisal from society, can make a person go through the full process of CME.

Preparation for CME

In this context it may not be presumptuous to consider preparing for CME to be one of the most important tasks of both basic medical training and specialist training. After all, the time span of CME is by far the longest period of learning.

Before discussing the role of basic medical training and specialist training in the preparation for CME, it might be profitable to consider some fundamental differences between the three stages of medical education concerning aims, teaching methods and organization.

In basic medical training, the aims and also the methods are determined by the government or the university. The students only have a marginal influence. There are special institutions with a permanent staff - medical schools - which provide for the teaching.

In specialist training, the aims are usually determined by the specialist associations or the universities. The curriculum is also usually set up by someone other than the trainee, although his influence on the actual contents of the study course is far greater than that of the medical student. In Sweden, the responsibility lies with the National Board of Health and Welfare.

In contrast, in CME the decisions on both aims and methods are made by the doctor, and there is no organization that has an overall responsibility. In short, during the process of medical training, students are required to develop from being a pupil who learns what is taught, to become independent professionals who make the decisions on all aspects of their own continuing education.

However, it is not enough to tell the students that as full-grown professionals they must analyse their learning needs, search out the road to knowledge themselves, and be prepared to cross the boundaries between different fields of learning. The methods of teaching must agree with this message. If not, the frustrated student is left with the duty of life-long learning, but with no instrument to carry it out. As this pedagogic contradiction is disastrous to motivation, it is necessary to discuss motivation and teaching methods together.

At present, there are two main types of medical schools: the Health Universities, such as Maastricht and Tromsö, and the traditional schools. Even if the traditional medical schools are changing, many still retain much of their old characteristics: the curriculum is divided into isolated subjects, reflecting almost exclusively the scientific content of medicine, disregarding social and humanistic aspects. The teaching is teacher-centred with minimal student influence regarding methods. The examinations aim at controlling that the student has grasped the facts of the course rather than its significance.

The Health Universities, by contrast, aim at integrating scientific, humanistic and social aspects of medicine: the teaching is multi-disciplinary and problem-oriented, leaving great freedom for students to find their own way to the desired knowledge. In examinations, understanding of the subject is more important than rote learning. The student is active, not passive.

This may be a crude review of some of the main differences between the traditional medical schools and the Health Universities but is only meant to illustrate the differences regarding their capacity to prepare the student for continuing professional education.

There are no doubts in my mind that many of the problems we have today with doctors who are unwilling, and unable, to participate in CME, have their roots in the traditional medical training. It must be a professional responsibility to support the development of medical schools in the direction of a teaching that is optimal with regard to CME - essentially that of the Health Universities. It is also the responsibility of the providers of vocational training to ensure that the new specialists have both the motivation to continue learning and the necessary knowledge and insights.

As in medical school, the way in which the training is organized conveys a more memorable lesson than any lecture on the ethics and techniques of CME. For instance, the new target-oriented specialist training system which will start operating in Sweden in 1992 is much better suited as a preparation for CME than the present one. It will require the trainee (preferably with the help of a trainer) to analyze his or her starting position and the goal of specialist training, and then conclude what this training should contain. This system is much more in line with CME than the present one, which only requires the trainee to complete a series of hospital and general practice appointments.

Specialist examinations could also be an instrument to promote CME. The first Swedish specialist examination of general practice, held in November 1989, required the candidates to list what medical journals and other scientific writings they had studied during their training. The organizers of the examinations have also discussed the possibility of including a group discussion on some topical, slightly controversial subject, such as the handling of moderate hypercholesterolemia or the treatment of chronic benign pain, where the candidates would be required to demonstrate that they are able to keep themselves adequately informed on current medical affairs.

The core of CME

The contents of continuing education may be considered under at least four headings: the doctors' need to maintain general medical knowledge; to develop their professional personality; to respond to the specific needs of the practice; and also to be used as a tool of change.

To keep abreast of the development of medical science doctors are expected to follow one or several medical journals, and to attend lectures. They are also expected to keep their medical practice up to date, and to co-operate with other health professionals. This implies educational efforts, sometimes of a massive kind, for example when a regional programme for diabetes is introduced.

By the phrase "develop the doctor's professional personality" is meant all endeavours to increase the doctor's intellectual, emotional and spiritual maturity, thus enhancing the capacity to perform as a doctor. Balint group work is an obvious example. The Danish 'twelve man groups' and different forms of peer review also belong to this category. What they have in common is that they all aim, in different ways, to increase the doctors' knowledge about themselves and their work. In my view, this is the most important branch of CME, just as the motivation to participate in CME is more important than having the technical learning skills.

Without knowing one's own strengths and weaknesses continuing education is likely to be haphazard and inefficient. Without at least the effort to assess objectively the doctor's practice, the educational activities chosen will reflect more the doctor's interests than his needs.

You may remember that Michael Balint presents his book 'The doctor, his patient, and the illness' as a report of a research project, and Balint group work, peer review and related activities are indeed close to research - the most sophisticated form of continuing education. What makes these forms of CME especially important is that general practice in its modern form is still a young speciality, with large areas as yet unchartered. Today, too much of our CME consists of fragments from other specialities, for the lack of sufficient material from our own. Investigations of individual practices may generate hypotheses of value for research and thus be the germ of new, more relevant knowledge.

Continuing education is also used as a tool of change. Health care systems change, usually through political decisions, and pedagogic efforts are commonly used to implement the decisions. The re-orientation of Sweden's primary health care towards team-work with other staff and co-operation with the social services would not have been achieved without educational efforts. In the important planning document 'The Swedish Health Services in the 1990s' continuing education is regarded as the most important instrument for the implementation of the changes proposed in the document.

The teaching projects of the Finnish health centres are another example of continuing education as a tool of change. These collaborative teaching projects, run by the

Department of General Practice and Primary Health Care at the University of Helsinki, are seen as a point of entry into developmental activities in the health centre.

Resources for CME

The problem of resources differs from one country to another, but there are some basic requirements for CME that are independent of the type of health care system. Most doctors would probably agree that a practice with several doctors provides an environment more favourable to CME than a single-handed practice. Not only is a larger practice more likely to maintain good library facilities and other practical aids to CME, but it will also make it easier to arrange leave to attend lectures and courses.

A more salient point is that in a group practice there is a chance to break the traditional isolation of general practice work. From 1978 to 1985, health centres with three or more doctors increased from 40 to 63 per cent in Sweden, and the number of centres with only one doctor decreased from 36 to 11 per cent and has gone down even further since then.

Time is the next prerequisite, and as time is money, it might be expedient to consider the two together. In principle, there are two main ways of paying the doctor in our countries. In the UK, Denmark and Iceland the general practitioner is self-employed, although paid mainly by the Health Authorities. In Sweden and Finland there are similar systems where the doctors are employed by the counties or the communities. It is interesting to note that in the UK, Denmark and Iceland there are provisions for CME in the contracts of the general practitioners, from five days per year for doctors in the UK to the very generous 15 days abroad every year for the Icelanders.

In Sweden and Finland, resources for CME as a rule have to come from the budget of the health centres, and thus compete with other needs. This makes it more difficult for general practitioners to travel to get to their CME unless they are prepared to pay their own way, or can find an outside sponsor. On the other hand, the Swedish-Finnish system is favourable to CME, which takes place in or near the health centre using local talent, and which does not require spending much ready money.

As both types of CME are desirable, the consequence is that doctors who are self-employed should work on making arrangements allowing them to spend time on local CME in working hours, whereas doctors who are employed by the community have to look after their interests regarding external CME.

It is characteristic of CME that it has no set organization to provide for it. In all our countries, the colleges of general practice and the medical associations seem to contribute greatly to CME as course organizers. The University Departments of general practice seem to play a much smaller role, except in Finland. This is unfortunate, as it is a natural part of the work of a University Department to spread its research results among practitioners, integrating the results in everyday work. But their resources are seldom sufficient to allow them to play a major role in CME. This is due to the fact that the size of the departments usually reflects the unimportance of general practice in the medical curriculum, and not its importance in the health care system.

The sticks and carrots of CME

The rewards of CME are usually insubstantial. It does not automatically bring a higher income, and the appreciation that a good doctor gets from colleagues and patients is not always directly proportional to the CME undertaken. It is difficult to construct a system of rewards that takes into account not only the quantity but also the results of the doctor's education. One would probably end up with something very much like the Fellowship by Assessment of the Royal College of General Practitioners, scrutinizing the doctor's entire professional activity.

CME probably has a lot to gain from having well-functioning systems for both punishing the failing doctor and rewarding the good one. The value of re-certification is more uncertain, not only on grounds of principle, but also on the grounds of effectiveness. If it is possible to get doctors to take part in CME only under the threat of losing their livelihood, one wonders if their motivation is sufficient for optimal learning.

On the other hand, the authorities that require re-certification must allow, and promote CME. A cooperation between these authorities and the medical associations could be very valuable, especially in a phase of development.

Conclusion

In order to improve the conditions for CME, we must work on many fronts. The most effective measures are probably those aiming at changing the teaching at the medical schools and the specialist training. Ideally, the three stages of medical training should function as one continuous educational process, where one important aim of the first two stages should be to prepare for the third one.

The university departments of general practice cannot play their proper role in CME, as long as their resources are inconsistent with the importance of general practice in the health care system. To strengthen general practice in medical schools would not only mean an improvement of the basic medical training but would also, through increased resources, strengthen the CME of general practitioners.

Regular reviews of the clinical work of medical students and trainees should be part of their training. This might diminish the anxiety which peer review and related activities seem to induce in doctors, and which is a main obstacle to effective CME, based on the doctor's true needs.

In order to run a good practice, funds for CME are as important as funds for premises or equipment. We must spell this out both to the authorities and to other groups of health professionals, with whom we compete for these funds.

Finally, let us not forget that to the true professional there is no enjoyment greater than feeling one's ability and understanding increasing over the years, making one's chosen profession more fascinating all the time - and that is what CME really is about.

STRATEGIES FOR CONTINUING EDUCATION

Professor Denis Pereira Gray - United Kingdom

Continuing Medical Education (CME)

Continuing medical education is a fascinating and complicated subject. I shall first consider its purpose and why it is so important and topical; secondly, review briefly the historical trends in its organization and provision; and finally look at current arrangements and especially its links with performance and audit and the way it is likely to develop in the immediate future.

In such a difficult and diffuse subject, I find in Rudyard Kipling's famous couplets a useful framework with which to analyse it:

> 'I keep six honest serving men,
> they taught me all I knew.
> Their names are "what" and "why" and "when"
> and "how" and "where" and "who"'.

1. Why?

First, we must clarify the purpose of continuing medical education. Strangely this is rarely stated. Its purpose is simple, namely to improve the care of the patient by improving the knowledge, skills and attitude of the general practitioner. Judged by this yardstick continuing education needs a complete relook, rethink and reorganisation.

2. What?

The question of what should be learned and what should be taught bedevils the subject. It is easy to say that doctors need to learn about new advances to help them keep up to date. But it is frequently said that an individual consultant or specialist can no longer keep up to date in his field. How then is it possible for the medical generalist to do the same across all the branches of medical practice?

The answer has to be a ruthless selection of priorities based on both wants and needs - a combination of what the individual wishes and needs, and what groups of generalists, working with and in touch with advancing specialist practices, perceive as their needs.

Performance/competency

What has never been clear, and is only now becoming clear, is how learning needs are to be identified. Here a major new advance in the last 25 years has been the increasing acceptance of the importance of performance, or as it is sometimes called, competency. Continuing medical education is being driven by issues of competency, both the failure of competency which may show up failures in education, and agreement about new competencies which always require new education.

As long ago as 1968, in an influential World Health Organisation document, 'the Competency-based Curriculum Development', McGaghie and Miller argued that the purpose of the curriculum should be simply to prepare doctors or medical students for the competencies that he or she would have to practise at the end of their education. A decade later, in 1979, the influential Cantor Lectures of the Royal Society of Arts in London emphasised the importance of what was then called 'education for capability'. This corresponds to the idea that the purpose of education is to improve performance or capability.

Now, at the end of the 1980s, this idea is reaching medical practice through the introduction of educational (medical) audit. This has long been a policy of the educational bodies in the United Kingdom, particularly the Royal Colleges, both generalist and specialist, but it is now to be introduced for all doctors in the National Health Service under the new Health Service Act of 1990.

The moment one accepts a competency-based approach to education then one is driven to accept the logic of defining in some way or other what competency of clinical care means. But this is extraordinarily difficult to do. No branch of specialist medicine has yet been able to define on paper exactly what competencies it expects of its practitioners. It is not possible, for example, to see the competency of a consultant surgeon or physician written down.

General medical practice, because it is both the oldest of the branches of medicine, on the one hand, and yet the newest to establish itself as an independent, clinical and academic discipline on the other, has all over the world accepted an educational approach to its development, and this has been true in the North American continent, in Australasia and in Europe. It was indeed general practitioners who were among the first to express their subject in terms of educational objectives (RCGP 1972).

But the objectives approach, so fashionable in the 1970s has become unfashionable in the 1980s. The reason is that it became counterproductive for expert working parties to list more and more objectives, which the long suffering student, trainee or doctor had to acquire. Clearly a new approach was needed, and that approach was to tackle the training triangle, 'Aims, Method and Assessment' (Pereira Gray 1977) at another point - the assessment point. Assessment is another word for performance, which again is another word for competency.

A major task for the Royal College of General Practitioners over the past decade, culminating as recently as June 1989, has been responding to the challenge of expressing in terms of competency the level of performance possible today for a general medical practitioner in the United Kingdom. How high can one go and still make it possible in practice? How can such competencies be measured? Who should do the measuring?

The College has tackled all these four issues and it has been one of the principal challenges of my Chairmanship to try to introduce a working model. In responding to competency we have simply agreed, first, that it should be measured in operational terms which are as unambiguous as possible; secondly, in order to fulfil the purpose of continuing education, that the criteria should be based entirely on the care of patients; and thirdly, that judgements on criteria cannot and should not be made by any single individual, but should be made corporately by the Royal College of General Practitioners. Next, since this is a constantly moving field, the principle should be accepted that the competence should be measured by peer review, and should be measured in the workplace, that is - where the patients are actually seen.

This major intellectual struggle to define 'the highest possible standards for general medical practice' culminated in the introduction of Fellowship by Assessment in our College in July 1989. Fellowship is the highest grade of membership of our College. This award can now be achieved by any member of the College of five years' standing who can now demonstrate objectively, before their peers in the setting of their own practices, that their standards for looking after patients, meet the very high standards determined by the College. Since it is so new, so far only six doctors have applied, but four of them have already been successful and have been admitted as fellows.

I believe that this new system represents a major innovation in continuing medical education because it states, for the first time, what high levels of competency or performance are. Of course the criteria are not perfect or even right, but the system provides for an annual review and a progressive adjustment in the light of experience of practice visiting, new research, and advancing professional practice.

3. When?

Continuing education for most of my professional lifetime has been a matter of reading and going to courses in the evenings and at weekends. Gradually, however, education is moving into the working week. Driven by patterns in industry, where training on the job, this has become the norm. The professions are responding, albeit slowly.

What is changing and changing fast is that the new technology is making it more possible and easier to access information where and when it is needed and particularly during the day's work. Any microcomputer suitably equipped with a modem can now access remote databases, not only in London but world-wide, through satellite technology. Similarly, the dramatic discovery of fax (the ordinary man's teleprinter) has provided a documentary equivalent to the telephone. We are now likely to look forward to faxes in our practices and the automatic receipt of information from colleagues in hospitals, and particularly in response to our educational needs, on a virtually instant basis.

4. Where?

Medicine in the first half of the twentieth century in the UK was dominated by the teaching hospital. As late as 1960 the advice to those doctors qualifying was simply to keep in touch with the teaching hospital because the teachers there at that time could not envisage original thought, original research or major developments in health services taking place outside their institutions.

It was however about the same time that the first major step towards the decentralisation of medical education began to emerge. First, and most important of all, the College of General Practitioners was founded in 1952. The Nuffield Conference of 1961 was crucial in bringing together those concerned with standards and education across the country, and under the stimulus of Sir George Pickering, an idea of peripheral postgraduate medical centres sprang up.

Information needs are being identified and met in a thousand different locations and the combined knowledge of mankind is being accessed and used in different ways at different times and in different places. The focal point now is no longer the ancient university and the collection of scholars, but the work setting where patients meet doctors, and the consulting room is now becoming the classroom in a new and dramatic way.

The impact of the new technology is essentially in the consulting room, and it is the arrival of the microcomputer on the doctor's desk that is its symbol. Already, for example, my microcomputer issues a bleep before a prescription is issued of any kind if the patient has any known allergy. I have already seen software demonstrations of interaction analyses which will remind doctors of any clinically important drug interaction before the prescription is issued. These developments have always been classified in the past as information technology, which of course they are. We also need to reclassify them in our minds as continuing education, because by constantly reminding the doctor at the time he or she needs reminding - in the consulting room - a new and very powerful educational process has been unleashed.

5. How?

The 'how' of continuing education will thus be information coming to the doctor in his or her practice and home, and increasingly by journals and books, by video, by disc and electronic transmission. Reflective analytical work is likely to continue to be on paper, whereas immediate factual needs will increasingly be met electronically. In countries like the Nordic countries, where doctors are working at great distances from academic centres and in the rural parts of the United Kingdom, entirely new and dramatic possibilities are unfolding for continuing education of a new quality and indeed of a new interest to the doctors concerned.

The human side of general practice is central. Face-to-face consultations are at the heart of our subject. Similarly in education face-to-face discussions and analyses will be at the heart of continuing education.

6. Who?

Finally a notable feature of continuing medical education has been the fact that only a minority of practitioners appear to avail themselves of it! Now, however, we face a new era in which the State will require on the one hand, and professional bodies will demand on the other, some participation in continuing educational activities by all of us. Medical audit is likely to be the mechanism by which some of this participation is achieved. Health authorities will soon be reviewing the reasons why some consultants and some general practitioners never go on courses at all. Questions may now be asked about the low users of continuing medical education whereas in the past all the focus has been on the high users.

Conclusion

In conclusion, I would like to suggest that 1990 is a key date in the history of continuing medical education for the medical generalist in many of the countries of Europe. If its central purpose is to improve the care of patients and if this is accepted, then the emphasis must now be on performance and competency, that is in determining what it is that doctors do for patients and how that can be improved.

The introduction of fellowship by assessment by means of a competencybased peer-review practice visit by the Royal College of General Practitioners is a turning point in the development of continuing education for general practitioners. This should provide, for the first time, a clear, written, nationally agreed target of good performance, and thus a clear direction for all College members of at least five years' standing, towards which to work. I see a general trend of decentralisation of education away from the old national academic centres of scholarship, away from the big teaching hospitals, via local postgraduate medical centres, into the practices themselves. These developments are being driven and encouraged by exciting new developments in information technology. Just as the horse has been replaced by the car and the plane, so information science is being transformed by modem access and the on-line search through the microcomputer. Fax will do for paper what the telephone has done for conversation.

Finally I see the ultimate in decentralisation will be when the original knowledge and the product of good clinical research in general practice itself starts to flow back into the world literature from general practices, and particularly from ordinary general practices, which will contribute increasingly to the research base of our discipline in the twenty-first century.
The whole history of general practice can be summarized as a struggle to obtain clinical and academic independence and a research-based, scientific basis of practice. Continuing medical education is about the dissemination and use of that knowledge and it is, I believe, about to take one of the biggest steps forward in its history.

References

Gray D J Pereira (1977) A System of Training. Occasional Paper 4. 2nd ed. London, Journal of Royal College of General Practitioners.

McGaghie W C, Miller G E et al. (1978) Competency-based Curriculum Development in Medical Education: an Introduction. Public Health Papers No. 68. Geneva, World Health Organization.

Royal College of General Practitioners (1972) The Future General Practitioner - Learning and Teaching. London, British Medical Journal.

Royal College of General Practitioners (1989) Fellowship by Assessment FBA1 London, Royal College of General Practitioners

Royal College of General Practitioners (1989) Medical audit in general practice. Statement by the Council of the RCGP. London, RCGP.

Royal Society of Arts (1979) Cantor Lectures. Journal of the Royal Society of Arts. London, RSA.

3. IMPLEMENTING POSTGRADUATE EDUCATION

Discussion points

'We have no money, therefore we have to think'.
Arne Ivar Østensen

Postgraduate education depends heavily on money, time and geography. For instance, in the UK there are large resources for vocational training but few for undergraduate or CME, which is reflected in the highly developed and structured vocational training course: in Scandinavia money for vocational training is less, but often time is more available for junior hospital doctors working only 40 hours a week and one night. Geography can be a major problem, the length of Norway is greater than the distance from Oslo to Rome.

Again we see trends in the diversity. UK and Norway both place great emphasis on teaching the teachers: in Finland the teaching is university based, but in Denmark there is no formal programme for teachers, which is a problem. There again we see a major difference between the UK and Scandinavia: do we need a tightly controlled system as in the UK, or can we trust the teachers? The latter is probably less reliable in terms of quality assurance, but allows greater diversity of response to individual needs, and is inevitable in large and sparsely populated countries.

All countries see the need for vocational training to lead on to continuing training. In Norway, five year re-accreditation for principals is based on the vocational training model: in the UK the educational advisers who manage vocational training are beginning to develop further training programmes for young general practitioners: in Denmark the young doctors respond to their isolation by forming 12 man groups.

Difficulties with the hospital component of vocational training are the rule. In Norway, a much larger component of training is now in general practice, but still involves long specialist modules: the Danes are arranging for the general practice component of vocational training to come early in order to pattern the young doctors' learning. In the UK the Royal College of General Practitioners (RCGP) is now jointly inspecting hospital posts. But closer cooperation between GP and hospital teachers must be the definitive solution. The six-monthly compulsory pre-registration time in general practice which applies in Denmark and Norway should help this understanding, but is disliked by many committed hospital doctors.

IMPLEMENTATION OF POSTGRADUATE TEACHING PROGRAMMES

by John Hasler

In the United Kingdom, the responsibility for the provision of postgraduate medical education rests, not with Universities, but with Regional Committees representing University and Health Authorities. There therefore is a division of responsibility between the education of medical students and of qualified doctors.

The two main components of postgraduate education - vocational training and continuing medical education (CME) - have been clearly identified. However, there is a third component sandwiched between the two known as higher training. This period, only operating in experimental forms in a few regions so far, is a time when young general practitioners can attend half-day release and residential courses that have a large emphasis on clinical and organizational management (1,2). As these courses become more widely established they will act as a bridge linking vocational training and CME.

For the purposes of this paper I shall examine each stage of postgraduate education in turn, and then draw some general conclusions.

Vocational Training

Although some schemes have effective teaching running throughout the hospital posts they are in the minority. Because the training based in hospital uses service posts and because of the increasing demands placed on the hospital service, especially in obstetrics and paediatrics, there has been considerable criticism of the lack of regular teaching by many consultants and the inability of trainees to attend half-day release courses (3). In any case, unless the trainees have had reasonable exposure to general practice, the main items on the trainees learning agenda are to do more with specialist than with general practice medicine.

The main educational activities occur during the general practice component, the bulk of which usually takes place in the third and final year. These activities are carried out in two main ways - regular tutorials and related activities in the teaching practice, and day release and other courses external to the practice.

The main underlying theme in vocational training is the need to make a major shift in the trainee's value system away from learning more and more clinical facts to the learning of fundamental behavioural skills, such as communication with patients, teamworking, auditing medical care and ways of keeping up to date.

This has two implications - much of the learning has to take place in small groups and the teachers need new skills in helping trainees to acquire these attributes.

Group Work

The importance of group work in vocational training has been documented (4) and now forms the basis for much activity in day release and residential courses. Unlike traditional learning in lectures, the participants are able to contribute equally and criticise each other more easily. They are able to observe interactive behaviour and discuss its interpretation. They are also able to solve problems as a group in the way they will need to do in their own practices.

Educating the Teachers

General practice has been the only medical specialty in the UK to look on education as a discipline in its own right to any great extent. Trainers in training practices are expected to have attended courses on educational method and to continue to develop their skills afterwards. Their practices are subject to regular inspection and re-inspection which is increasingly rigorous (5).

Some trainers have found this new world exciting and have made major advances whilst others have found it difficult. At Oxford we have been experimenting with a number of ways of helping the trainers of which two deserve a mention.

Following work done in the early eighties by Pendleton et al (6) a consultation skills course is now provided regularly. It lasts for three days, is residential and helps doctors to understand the need for clear objectives during consultations. Each participant learns how to assess consultations on videotape, conducts a consultation with specially trained actors in front of a small group and is finally given the opportunity to practise giving feedback to his colleagues on their performance.

The second residential course is on educational method, emphasising the principles of adult learning. It enables participants to evaluate tutorials on videotape and gives help in maintaining momentum throughout the training period whilst developing educational objectives through a series of stages.

Using the Primary Health Team

Most of the teaching done in training practice tutorials is done by the GP Trainer or one of his partners. Increasingly, it is being recognised that nursing and managerial members of the team have important contributions to make.

Higher Training

During the last three years at Oxford we have been experimenting with higher training courses for young general practitioners. At the beginning we taught according to subject areas, but it soon became clear that what was needed was the opportunity to develop skills. Our most recent model, which seems to be successful, comprises three stages.

The first is clinical management when the participants identify strategies and mechanisms of coping with clinical problems, especially long term ones. Next, operational management is examined and the needs of the primary health team in effective organisation. Finally, participants look at their own personal and professional growth.

The original course was a series of half-day sessions spread over two years. It was found, however, that taking three hours out from a busy practice commitment did not work particularly well. The group members took a long time to get to know each other and the amount of work some of them were able to achieve was limited.

The model now adopted is a series of three 2-3 day residential modules spread over one year with half-day release sessions spread between. This has made it possible for much more work to be done in a relaxed setting and for members to undertake a number of projects during the year. They are also able to visit each other's practices in a structured fashion which has been extremely popular.

Continuing Medical Education

Turning to CME, there are two broad aims of all programmes. One is to contrive to develop generic skills in GPs who may have had insufficient grounding in vocational or higher training. The other is to provide updating.

Updating

Traditional methods have largely involved lectures and presentations, usually by specialists. The objectives for such activities are usually implicit and little evaluation has taken place. The introduction of new arrangements for CME for GPs with stricter criteria for accreditation will hopefully mean that relevance and standards will improve.

For example in the Oxford Region objectives now have to be stated and an appropriate GP involved before course approval is given. Some attempt at evaluation is required. We hope in time that we will be able to demonstrate increasing sophistication and effectiveness in updating mechanisms.

Further Skills Development

Several of these important skills have already been mentioned - consultation, teamworking, audit and other aspects of management.

In the field of management a number of different courses are now being provided in the Oxford Region. A course in interviewing and selection techniques has been developed where participants learn how to conduct structured interviews in depth for the purposes of selecting partners, staff and trainees. Each participant goes through the procedures on videotape in front of a tutor and group members and is introduced to the concept of personality testing. In the field of prevention a course involving mini primary care teams of doctors, nurses, health visitors and practice nurses has been designed in conjunction with the Health Education Authority. In the light of experience with the first few courses, it has become clear that the main gain is largely to do with effective teamworking for any purpose, rather than merely prevention.

In parallel with these developments locally appointed facilitators, usually nurses, have been appointed in many districts in the region to work directly with individual practices to further the progress towards effective prevention. In one health district, the project has been so successful that nearly every practice in the district is now involved.

With the introduction of compulsory medical audit for hospital doctors and general practitioners from April 1991, we are currently exploring ways of providing education both for the supervisory committees and individual practices which are likely to reflect the methods already described for other subjects.

Conclusions

It can be seen that ways of implementing postgraduate education provision are developing in an exciting way. It has become clear that the tutors, once they are familiar with how to lead small groups, are almost interchangeable between one course and another. Frequently, new tutors go through a course themselves, then being selected to act as tutor next time.

The problem of appointing local GP tutors to coordinate and plan district activities such as regular lectures and symposia has been increasingly worrying. At the moment there is no agreed funding system for those doctors and their appointments are precarious or non-existent in some places.

Apart from this difficulty, the future of postgraduate education for general practice in the UK looks bright.

References

1. Royal College of General Practitioners (1987) The Front Line of the Health Service. RCGP London. Report from General Practice No 25, Para 4.34.

2. Higher Professional Training (Oxford Region in preparation).

3. Reeve, H and Bowman, A (1989) Hospital training for general practice: views of trainees in the North Western Region. Br Med Jnl, 298, 1432-4.

4. Gray, D & P (1977) A System of Training for General Practice. RCGP Occasional Paper 4, pp16-17.

5. Schofield, T P C and Hasler, J C Approval of trainers and training practices in the Oxford Region. Br Med Jnl 1984, 288: 538-540, 612-614, 688-689.

6. Pendleton, D A, Schofield, T P C, Tate, P H L and Havelock, P B (1984) The Consultation. An Approach to Learning and Teaching. Oxford University Press. General Practice Series No 6.

4. TEACHING METHODS FOR GENERAL PRACTICE

Discussion points

'Knowledge about a subject is what is left
when we have forgotten all the information'.
Claes Kjær

'I taught my tiger to whistle'.
'But I can't hear anything'.
'I said I taught it, I didn't say it learned'.
Jamie Bahrami

Once again, in this section, we see the emphasis placed by the UK/Nordic group on adapting the teaching and learning to the learner's needs. The power of learning only occurs when the information transmitted is 'personalized' by the learner, and so appreciated as relevant to his understanding and his needs. How then can we discover needs? David Metcalfe suggested that learning needs can be expressed as a Venn diagram (below).

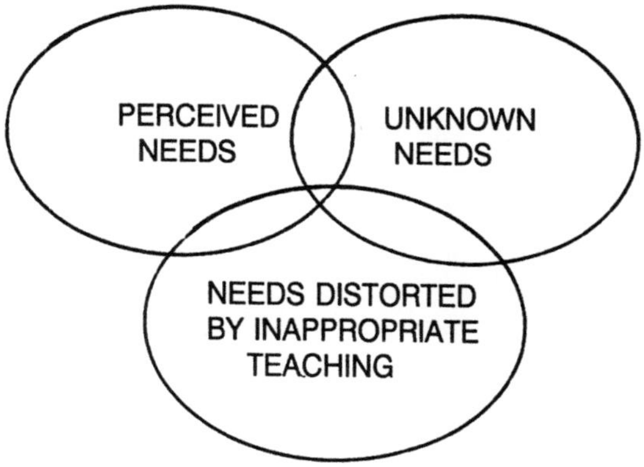

In order to move from 'unknown' to 'perceived' while avoiding distortion, we must enable learners to self-direct, perhaps best by using problem-based teaching. Concern was expressed that such teaching may leave gaps in knowledge, but we were assured that at Tromsö, one of the new universities using this method, students have more factual knowledge and are better at problem solving. Even when covering the core of knowledge and skills it appears that learners who direct their own programme feel a possession of the curriculum and develop their own set of values while learning.

As a result of this conclusion the role of assessment returns to the fore. Learning, especially at junior levels, tends to be examination-led: this is the opposite of self-direction. Assessment is essential in order to determine need, and formative assessment must be central to developing the appropriate teaching methods. We must make more formative assessment available at all levels. In turn, such formative assessment can provide career guidance, and support for young doctors during the hospital phase of training - both are areas often neglected throughout medical teaching.

Perhaps most important of all is the facility for students to assess and develop their values. We need a curriculum to develop aims and programmes for teaching, but it must not be so structured as to deny students the facility to develop their own values. We have to resolve the paradox of self-direction and curriculum. By self-direction the curriculum can be assessed, personalised and internalised, and the student can begin to feel possession of his own learning. Perhaps values is a less pejorative word than attitudes in the triad of 'knowledge, skills and values', and values can only be developed not taught. Scandinavian countries, with less structured primary care teams, less structured education systems and apparently more time, seem to be able to teach the UK a good deal about this.

TEACHING METHODS FOR GENERAL PRACTICE

Claes Kjær - Denmark

On information, knowledge, and experience.

In postgraduate training, the aim is to teach the participants all the important issues within our profession. We do our utmost, and yet it often seems as if our efforts have no effect. Sometimes, however, the results are surprisingly good, and we do not know exactly how we succeeded in doing the miracle that occurs when information becomes useful knowledge, and when new experience can be linked to experience already achieved and become a constructive unit.

Education and training must be considered a process enabling us to deal with our own everyday, professional life. Everyday life does not consist of well-defined facts and regulations, but of our episodic memory from earlier situations we have mastered.

In postgraduate training of general practitioners, we often use instructors who are experts within their field. The everyday life of such experts (and of the participants) is not governed by formal logic and external rules. Instructors and participants each possess personal knowledge. In a teaching situation, the instructor organizes his personal knowledge in separate and well-defined elements. In other words, he passes information.

This kind of communication used by the instructor - the transformation of personal knowledge into well-defined information - can be illustrated by direct contemplation of a person's face compared to the same face built in high-resolution graphics on a computer screen. At first glance, the two faces may seem identical, but at a closer look, we find that the face on the screen actually consists of small isolated points whose position and colour are carefully defined by individual bits of information.

This means that when we communicate our personal knowledge, it becomes public information whereby something is lost. Within the field of perception psychology, we use the term 'gestalt', which is defined as integrated units containing more than the mere sum of the individual elements they consist of. On the basis of this definition, it can be said that knowledge is organized in gestalts and, therefore, always contains more than just the sum of information which can be communicated.

It is important to be aware of the difference between knowledge gestalts and individual information, as these are two dimensions, both indispensable in any kind of education. Thus, learning something is not just a matter of gathering as much information as possible about a chosen subject, it is also an exercise in forming a coherent gestalt of knowledge about the subject. To put it simply, knowledge about a certain subject is what is left when we have forgotten all the information. And once we possess this knowledge gestalt, we can easily find the necessary information when needed in a specific situation.

To concentrate education on passing information in an information technological society is, therefore, not a wise strategy to follow when we want to modernize education and training. Knowledge is information which has been through a process whereby the information is personalized. The training situation consists, therefore, of a generalizing phase, a transmission phase, and a personalization phase. As mentioned, the generalizing phase is the passing of information, the transmission phase is the 'digesting' phase, and the personalization phase is the most important one in order to make information into useful knowledge. The personalization phase often takes place in a social situation and in a socio-cognitive conflict within the person or participant during discussion, dialogue, and constructive antagonism. Hereby information can 'melt' into the person and become part of that person.

In most teaching situations, the personalization phase is often lacking, although this is the phase to concentrate on in the continuing medical education of general practitioners. The important part of learning - the personalization phase - is a painful process which the instructor and the participants naturally seek to avoid, resulting in a reduced learning effect.

Methods

In continuing medical education, I have personal experience in using methods which, in many ways, ensure that the participants go through the painful process of learning and thus experience the satisfaction of being able to use what they have learned in a practical way. The methods are:

- Problem oriented learning;
- Exchange of experience;
- Project oriented work.

None of these methods are, of course, a paradigm of how instruction should be, but all the methods are very different from lecturing as an instruction method.

1. Problem Oriented Learning

Here the group - or the groups - works with a theme which has been decided upon beforehand. Problem oriented learning is divided into various steps:

A. Concept Definition
The group ensures that all participants understand and agree on the content of the concepts.

B. Problem Definition
The aim here is to make the group understand the contents of the problem, and it is decided which problems to deal with.

C. **Problem Analysis**
Here a brain-storm on the problem can be practical as well as an analysis of the problem, enabling the participants to realize if they need to gather further information in order to understand the problem.

D. **Final Formulation of Learning Needs**
Here the group decides and agrees upon what further information is needed and what skills the group wishes to obtain within the field.

E. **Obtaining Knowledge in relation to Learning Needs**
Here the group decides how to achieve knowledge and skills in the best way and how best to take advantage of resources and resource persons.

F. **Evaluation of Achieved Knowledge**

2. Exchange of Experience

Experience - which is part of the knowledge gestalts - develops when we reflect on the impressions we get cognitively, affectively and physically. As compared to information, experience is what we get when we act - it is the result of an act we take part in. Experience is personal and has an authentic quality. It is concrete, whereas, as mentioned, information is abstract and general. Experience is connected with acting or the wish to achieve something, and it develops in the area between expectations based on previous experience and the actual results of an act. Thus, the development of experience is attached to personal, creative acting.

In a teaching situation, experience-pedagogic instruction may take place, for example by letting the participants describe part of their own work, discuss this, learn from each other's good sides and make proposals to/for each other about changes or improvements.

3. Project Oriented Work

Project oriented work entails the participants receiving a number of project titles from the instructor, which they themselves discuss in the groups where they decide how to handle the problem, and decide which information is necessary in order to proceed with the project and make use of existing resource persons or other kinds of resources - literature, equipment, surrounding society, etc.

Example

As an example, I would like briefly to describe a course I held for physicians from various specialities, including general medicine, in 1989. The course was titled 'The Doctor as a Teacher'. The aim of the course was to improve the postgraduate instructor's teaching by giving the participants new knowledge about the importance of teaching methods in order to achieve successful learning, and to let the participants discuss, evaluate, and test the teaching methods in skill training within the methods of lecturing, panel discussion, and personal and group supervision.

On the first evening of the course, a video tape with authentic lectures was presented to the groups which then discussed the good and less good qualities of the lectures and evaluated the methods of the lecturers, including the audiovisual equipment used.

The following day, the participants, in groups, presented a 10 min. lecture which they had prepared beforehand. Hereafter the groups discussed and shared the experience on lecturing as teaching method. All lectures were video taped and one was selected from each group to be presented in plenary, where more general problems would be pinpointed.

The course concluded with role play dealing with supervision situations based on the participants' own experience from their profession. In the arrangement of the course we ensured that exchange of experience, project oriented work, presentation of projects, and the evaluation phase were used in the teaching process.

As the course proceeded, an increasing restlessness among the participants could be noted, and in the critical middle of the course one of them made a statement about his views of the course. He said that when arranging courses, it is important not to have problems with the FOMP. The Form was wrong. The useless group work was intolerable considering what information one could expect to receive in order to become a better teacher. The Organization of the course was wrong. The relation between working hours and the result was not reasoned out. The project work as a working Method was reprehensible and useless. All in all, the instructors should go back and reconsider the Planning of their courses.

I thought a lot about what went wrong during that course and, of course, my first reaction was that in spite of everything there are still doctors who prefer to be informed, instead of going through painful learning methods as those described above.

Three months later, we sent out an evaluation questionnaire, specially with a view to receiving information as to whether some of the participants had used what they might have learned during the course. To my big surprise, the critical participant wrote the following:

> "Much in spite of myself, I must admit that I have changed my teaching considerably after the course, but that was not because of the instructor!"

In summary, it is important to remember the difference between information and knowledge. We must remember that the transmission phase and the personalization phase are what we are aiming at in our teaching in continuing medical education, and we must consider teaching and education as part of individual development. We must learn, through exchange of experience, to take advantage of intuition and to accept the benefits of irrationality. I, for my part, still consider a successful learning process a miracle!

TEACHING METHODS FOR GENERAL PRACTICE

Sirkka Keinänen-Kiukaanniemi - Finland

'Good teaching is like an elephant:
it is difficult to define, but
you notice it when you meet one'.

L. Kalevi Korhonen

Introduction

The year 1988 was a significant one for teaching in the University of Oulu for two reasons. Firstly, responsibility for specialist training in general practice, the largest field of specialization in Finland, was transferred from the authority of the National Board of Health to the universities in that year and secondly that year had been designated a special year of teaching at the University. It is true indeed, at least in Finnish universities, that the activities needed for the development and evaluation of teaching methods always remain in the shadow of other activities, especially of research.

For decades few changes have happened in traditional under-graduate medical education in Finland although changes in society have created new needs. The undergraduate education has remained the same in its structure, but the amount of knowledge included in it has enormously increased. Now, there seems to be a gap between the goals of undergraduate education and its content (1).

Remedying this gap between the basic medical education and the professional needs of general practitioners is the most important challenge for vocational training of general practice in Finnish medical faculties at present.

Teaching methods for general practice

I will define method as follows: 'A teaching method refers to the means by which educational services are arranged and implemented; it is an entity of arrangements by which the person responsible for teaching can direct the learners to achieve their learning goals in the course of a teaching process'.

This definition includes the idea that teaching methods cannot be discussed in the absence of teaching goals. In other words, the goals determine the methods. Already the goals, framework and structure of training programmes have been created in the five medical faculties according to the recommendations given by the national Working Group on Specialization in General Practice (2). The next step must be the development of appropriate methods for achieving the goals of education.

A good teaching method is one which results in learning. It is not sensible to talk about teaching unless we talk about learning at the same time. Learning and teaching are not the same thing. Plenty of learning goes on without there being any teaching, and not all teaching necessarily leads to the desired learning. Therefore it would be more appropriate to concentrate more on learning than on teaching methods.

Learning by teaching

Although learning and teaching are not the same thing there is one point where teaching and learning coincide; when you teach you also learn. When you teach you have to consider your own ways of working, your methods and the validity of the subject matter in a quite different way as when working alone. Participation in undergraduate teaching is a good method of learning general practice for future key persons.

How do adults learn?

When we talk about specialization or vocational training for general practice we are clearly dealing with adult education which differs from that of children and young people in many respects. The principles of adult education do not necessarily apply in the undergraduate teaching situations, because the maturing process from adolescence to mature adulthood has not yet finished in young students. Studying at this early stage often is externally motivated and a major part of this basic education is compulsory and its content strictly defined. The main aim of the students is often to pass the coming examinations. This easily leads to 'superficial learning' rather than a profound understanding of the topics concerned.

The basic principles of adult learning are the following:

1. Adult learning is self-initiated, self-motivated, self-managed and self-evaluated.

2. Different people prefer different kinds of learning experiences.

3. Adult learning is most effective when it is related to a perceived need.

4. Adults tend to build on what they already know.

Self-directed learning in adult education

Many studies concerned with adult education have shown that the best method is 'self-directed learning'. There is convincing evidence that people who take the initiative of learning into their own hands learn more and better than people who remain passive, and that they are also better at using and retaining the knowledge and skills they have learned. Self-directed learning is in harmony with the natural psychological development of the human being. The need for independence, first from the control of one's parents and then from teachers and other adults, increases as one grows up, and dependence is replaced by a need to act independently, free of such control.

The principle of self-directed learning is that the learning process is based on learning needs and the requirements of the student, which are determined according to his work and his initial situation. There are four phases in the self-directed learning process:

1. Determining the content areas of the work
2. Determining the learning needs
3. Drawing up the curriculum
4. Evaluating the learning outcomes

Self-directed learning seems well suited for the training of specialists in general practice, but this does not mean studying alone or totally unsupervised.

Self-directed learning at Oulu University

The method has particular advantages for vocational training in the University of Oulu. The Oulu Faculty of Medicine is the northernmost of the five faculties in Finland and geographically serves approximately half the country. The number enrolled for further training is 80 at present, but will soon rise to over 100. These people live all over Northern Finland, so that the density of trainees in the region is 1/1000 sq Km. The Department of General Practice has only three assistant teachers and one Professor, and most of their time is spent on implementing basic education. It therefore seems almost impossible for these four people to satisfy all the educational needs of the candidates for vocational training. The principle of self-directed learning thus seems a natural and suitable method against this background.

The method has been applied in the following way. The candidates for training are convened for an 'opening seminar' to plan the course of their further education. The students meet together in groups at the initial stage to define and examine the content of their own work, its special features and the knowledge, skills and occupational development needed for it. This is also an excellent opportunity for them to study the professional values and attitudes of a general practitioner.

In the second phase the students themselves determine their learning needs with respect to both content and tasks. In other words, they go through the whole content of the work and the fields to be studied and identify those areas in which they already feel that they are competent and those areas in which they need further information and training. This analysis is made in written form by each candidate personally, and it is discussed individually with an instructor.

In the third phase the students draw up a curriculum based on the learning needs observed and existing training alternatives. A certain number of positions for general practice training are available in both hospitals and health centres in each part of the region. The needs revealed in the opening seminars make it possible to plan and coordinate the use of these positions. Each person plans a syllabus for the time available and makes proposals regarding its implementation, including both service in various wards and outpatient departments and theoretical courses in the subjects required. Each syllabus is gone through in detail in the opening seminars and possible gaps are examined. At the end of the seminar the participants may arrive at the conclusion that not all the training needed is available, and an alternative plan has to be drawn up. A fruitful interaction and discussion arises between the instructors and candidates. The training can be planned with the needs of the candidates in mind, but fields which the instructor regards as important can also be included, and a similar balance is achieved in the theoretical courses. The instructor or those responsible for the teaching are also expected to arrange courses and satisfy training needs which cannot be taken care of in any other way.

This method has already been used in the University of Tampere by Professor Mauri Isokoski. He now has experience of arranging these opening seminars for about 100 trainees. They have produced study plans with contents that show a clear emphasis on large clinical specialties. The failure of the trainees themselves to realize the importance of general practice topics to a sufficient extent is probably due to the fact that no proper professional identity for general practitioners has yet been formed, because conscious training began only when responsibility was transferred to the universities.

Learning by experience

The way in which general practitioners learn best, in a self-directed context as well as by other methods, is by experience. All experience is learning. But experiences can be used in different ways for this purpose and it should be possible to increase their use during the learning process. Learning by experience can be a planned part of the training system, or it can take place almost unconsciously through everyday events. Learning by experience could be promoted in future by arranging weekly case meetings in which each student in turn presents problematic situations or patient cases.

Summary

In Finland the implementation of vocational training is a major challenge for universities. Goals and a basic framework for the training programme have been created, and now it is the time of developing teaching methods to achieve the goals.

When choosing the teaching methods for vocational training in general practice the principle of adult education as well as local circumstances should be taken into account. The responsibility for learning is on the shoulders of trainees and the contents of teaching and learning are derived from the learners' needs and from the contents of work. The role of teacher is to stimulate the motivation and to create the circumstances for learning. The most important goal is to create a positive attitude towards continuing medical education and life-long learning.

References

1. Kumpusalo, E, Mattila, K, Virjo, I, Neittaanmki, L, Kataja, V, Kujala, S, Jskelinen, M, Luhtala, R and Isokoski, M. Medical education and the professional needs of young physicians in Finland. To be published 1990.

2. Working group on Organization of specialist training of general practice in Finland. Ministry of Education 1987.

3. Knowles, M. Self-directed learning. A guide for learners and teachers. Cambridge Adult Education, USA. 1975.

TEACHING METHODS IN GENERAL PRACTICE

Jamie Bahrami - United Kingdom

Teaching and learning in general practice can be made more stimulating and enjoyable if we use a variety of teaching methods. In this section, I would like to consider some of the appropriate methods that we can use in Vocational and Continuing Medical Education. But, first, we must remind ourselves of some of the well- known principles of teaching.

Principles of Teaching

1. Educational Paradigm

To talk about methods without first considering the educational paradigm, 'aims, method and assessment' is an impossible proposition. The first phase in the planning of any educational activity must be clear definitions of aims and objectives.

2. Subject Matter

The subject can, to a certain extent, determine the most appropriate method of teaching. Teachers must not believe that anything can be taught and learnt by only one particular method. For instance, it seems unreasonable to use group meetings as the best means of teaching a practical skill such as joint injection or minor surgery. This is best taught by demonstration and then performance by the learner under supervision.

3. Elements of Learning

In adult education, there are many crucial elements which will have to be considered by teachers at all times:-

- The learner must be made responsible for his own education and encouraged towards the principle of self-directed learning.

- Educationalists refer to mutuality in learning, ie the learner has to be a 'giver' as well as a 'getter' of information.

- Feedback/evaluations are essential elements of any educational activity. Medical teachers may go through the whole exercise of collecting the feedback data but then take very little notice of the reactions of the participants. This is a complete waste of time.

- The teacher should, regardless of the type of teaching method, always pay attention to good preparation for any educational session. For instance, the physical environment should be as conducive to learning as possible.

Teaching Methods: 1. Lectures

Currently, in the educational circle of general practice, the lecture is seen as an outdated and ineffective method of teaching. Paradoxically, the evidence suggests that, as far as the learners are concerned, it is by far the most frequent and popular form of continuing medical education. The real reason for the success or failure of a lecture largely depends on whether or not it is the most appropriate form of teaching for a particular subject.

It is commonly acknowledged that lectures can fulfil the following aims:-

- Provide the learner with an overview of the subject
- Direct the learner's course of study and thought
- Convey specific areas of facts and information

Lectures can be used much more imaginatively than they commonly are. For instance, in the context of vocational training, a lecture can be based on the problems and issues the trainees/trainers have been asked to bring to the session. In this way, the lecturer can respond to the specific educational needs and difficulties of the group. Another exciting way of using lectures is to start the session by a multiple choice question paper, modified essay question paper or, indeed, any other trigger material which would help the group to focus its attention upon the content of the lecture.

2. Group Learning

Over the past decade or so, group learning has become the clear battle-cry of every avant-garde teacher of general practice in the United Kingdom. In many circles group learning is considered to be the only form of effective education, although there is little evidence to substantiate this claim.

Like any other method of teaching, group learning can be effective if used properly and disastrous if not. A teacher, before choosing group learning, must be absolutely clear about his aims for the session. The three acknowledged aims for group learning are:-

- Application of knowledge (cognitive skills)
- Development of thinking and oral skills
- Development of appropriate attitudes

There are also some subsidiary aims, eg self-understanding, uncovering covert attitudes, developing leadership skills, establishing an opportunity for comparative analysis of work and attitude.

The essential factor to ensure success in group work is a group leader with the necessary leadership skills who can maintain the group and focus its work on the issues that come before it. The group leader should always be chosen with care and certainly prior to the date of the activity. Selecting anyone as a group leader on the day of the course and then providing him with a list of instructions on how to conduct the group work will lead to disaster. It is a myth that for group work all you need to do is put a few doctors in a room, lock the door and wait for something magical to happen.

3. Role Play

This is one of the most valuable and, at the same time, under-used methods of teaching. Although it can be used with great success in management training, eg teaching of teamwork, decision making and interviewing skills, its real value lies in unravelling emotional and personal dilemmas that are experienced by individuals in the group.

There are two methods of using role play. First, the teacher can devise a scenario which is handed out to the members of the group to act. The second, but more effective way, is for the members of the group to role play their own problems. This is particularly appropriate when the problem presented has no clear solution. The teacher's role in such a situation is to provide sufficient flexibility within the session not only to realize the aims but also help to resolve emotional upheavals that such an experience can cause.

4. One-to-One Teaching

Every training practice in the UK is now expected to provide a minimum of three hours a week protected time for teaching. During this period, the trainer and trainee, away from the hustle and bustle of the practice, retire to their common-room/library for an hour or so of quiet discussion.

Surprisingly, this form of 'cosy' teaching activity often causes a great deal of anxiety for both the trainer and the trainee. For the trainer, because of not knowing what and how to teach and for the trainee of the fear of having to endure another mini lecture. There are also difficulties when the trainer fails to keep the trainer:trainee relationship on a colleague to colleague rather than teacher to pupil basis. Consequently, the trainee is put in a very passive and defensive position which is difficult to explore. Another serious problem associated with this form of teaching is the 'collusion' that evolves between the trainer and trainee not to upset each other. And, as a result, the whole teaching and learning becomes superficial and non-threatening.

How then should we plan our one-to-one teaching? As an educational principle, it is undoubtedly better to relate the knowledge and skill taught to the practical experiences of the trainee (experiential learning). In this instance, case discussion assumes supreme importance. However, to make full use of its potential, it must be informative, participative and, above all, enjoyable. In this way, the case discussion should be aimed at uncovering the individual and personal difficulties and attitudes of the trainee. It should encourage decision making, performance review, familiarity with the literature and even project work. The following might be a useful summary of the methods that could form the basis of one-to-one teaching:-

Random case analysis, case presentation, problem case discussion, critical reading, project work, consultation, examination of the trainee's log book, formative assessment, personal difficulties and performance review.

Conclusions

It is clear that no single method of teaching is superior to any other and, as teachers, we should attempt to make use of different methods for different purposes.

To plan an effective teaching session, it is generally agreed that the following steps should be followed:-

1. Define clearly the aims, stating precisely what the learner is expected to learn.
2. Determine and plan what prior learning is required.
3. Design a sequence of learning which will make the session lively and effective.
4. Identify the most appropriate methods for learning and use more than one method if at all appropriate.
5. Assess the learning intermittently and at the end.
6. As a teacher, show enthusiasm, excitement and enjoyment throughout the session.

Further Reading

1. Bligh, D 1972 What's the use of Lectures? Penguin, Harmonsworth
2. Powell, L S 1973 Lecturing. Pitman Publication, London.
3. Brown, G 1982 The Medical Teacher. Churchill Livingstone, Edinburgh
4. Colyer, J Medical Education as Abuse. Br Med Jnl v 299 1989 pp 1408-1409
5. Bion, W 1961 Experiences in Group Work. Tavistock Publications

5. ASSESSMENT IN ACTION

Discussion points

'To the student we owe formative assessment,
to the patient we owe summative assessment,
to society we owe evaluation of their services'.
David Metcalfe

The need for formative assessment has been well argued throughout each stage of this report. Without it, students, be they junior or established, cannot assess their needs or develop further educational aims. Each country is, in its way, moving towards formative assessment. In the UK there is 'What sort of doctor?' and the development of 'Fellowship (of the RCGP) by assessment'. The Norwegians describe a centralized project for assessing the value and results of small group CME work. The Swedes are beginning to offer assessment during their modular multidisciplinary courses. The Finns are starting a project of going into health centres to set up quality assurance programmes in practice.

Summative assessment is much more difficult. In Norway, for instance, summative assessment ends at the end of basic medical training: whereas in the UK, Donald Irvine describes a detailed and rigorous programme of summative assessment after vocational training. Several countries are now looking at re-accreditation, currently required in Norway but only on the basis of attendance, not of examination. There is also a project in Northern Sweden, but it is voluntary. The programme of re-accreditation is seen as stimulating the doctors and reassuring for the public. But there is a view that re-accreditation is an acknowledgement of professional failure to maintain standards.

Formative and summative assessment are, then, liable to be contradictory. As expressed by Metcalfe, formative assessment requires validity, summative assessment reliability. The medical establishment has traditionally favoured reliability over validity, but this will not do for general practice. This paper has repeatedly emphasized the importance of values, and valid assessment is necessary to reinforce this. Invalid assessments - however reliable - may constrain freedom to develop - 'assessment may severely limit your growth'.

There is also a view that continuing assessment may be seen as threatening, and so be undesirable, especially in under-doctored areas. But the key must be the distinction between formative and summative assessment: lowering standards was never the answer to revitalising the profession.

Programmes of performance review and assessment will continue: they will be exploratory and varied. Summative assessment is usually voluntary - and should remain so at least until we are more expert in it.

EVALUATION OF GENERAL PRACTITIONERS' SPECIALTY TRAINING IN NORWAY

Bjørn Oscar Hoftvedt and Steinar Westin - Norway

Introduction

General practice has been recognised as an independent specialty in Norway since 1985. The Norwegian Medical Association (NMA) has structured a five year postgraduate training programme. An essential element of the educational programme is two years of organised group work. The trainees take part in local groups led by a trained tutor. Each group consists of from 2-10 general practitioners practising in the same area.

In January 1986 the first 38 groups were established. The groups were spread all over Norway and it was impossible for the specialty committee to monitor (or control) them. The committee, however, felt that they needed to know how the educational programme worked in practice; did the groups meet regularly, what did they discuss, did they work according to the programme described in the Educational Handbook (1), were the participants still friends after one year of close collaboration, or had some groups broken up?

The specialty committee therefore decided to evaluate the programme and an evaluation committee was appointed by the Norwegian Medical Association. The committee's mandate was to evaluate the whole programme of specialty training, but concentrate particularly on the group work of the first 38 groups.

In this article we will discuss the evaluation methods we used, their strengths and weaknesses compared with other ways of evaluation. A summary of two of the evaluation studies will also be presented.

The evaluation committee

In Norway the Ministry of Health and Social Affairs has delegated the responsibility for the specialty training to NMA. Within NMA each specialty has its own committee. The evaluation committee consisted of two members representing the specialty committee, one trainer, one trainee, one member of the College of General Practitioners, one member of the Association of General Practitioners and one from the secretariat of NMA.

Values in evaluation

A possible criticism is that two members of the specialty committee, which was responsible for the educational programme, also took part in the evaluation of it. These two persons had the opportunity to influence the interpretation and the presentation of the results of the evaluation. However, the main objective of the evaluation was not to conduct a rigorous, objective study, but to provide the specialty committee with sufficient feedback to improve the education. Therefore it was of great importance to have an open communication and a good relationship between the two committees. The two members serving on both the committees could also possibly contribute to the implementation of the results of the evaluation.

The outcome approach of evaluation

External evaluation also has a tendency to emphasise the control aspect of evaluation (summative evaluation). The task is to define objective measurable aims and then study the educational programme in order to find out whether they are fulfilled. If the results of such an evaluation show that the educational programme has not fulfilled its aims, the conclusion is usually that the programme has failed. This way of evaluating educational programmes does not describe whether the programme has achieved other beneficial results than those planned. The outcome approach is not usually concerned about why the programme did not succeed, and so the results are not very useful for directing any improvements of the programme.

The qualitative approach of evaluation

Researchers who intend to evaluate the outcome of an educational programme are usually influenced by research methods developed for the natural sciences (2). They demand random sampling, measurable variables, control group design and use of sophisticated statistical methods (3).

The qualitative or intuitive approach, however, tries to investigate the process in order to acquire knowledge about how the plans are carried out. They are not uninterested in the outcome, but they are more concerned about why something eventually goes wrong. The most common methods are unstructured interviews, observation, diaries or other written reports.

This approach has been criticised as being too subjective. David Terpstra (4) reviewed 52 articles on evaluation of organization development interventions and found that those evaluations that had applied less methodological rigour tended to be biased towards positive findings. Only five articles reported uniformly negative findings, and all these five studies had a rigorous methodological approach. However, if the main purpose of the evaluation is to improve the educational programme, it is not satisfactory only to report negative or positive findings.

Planning of the evaluation of the specialty training of general practitioners in Norway

When planning evaluation both structure, process and outcome of educational events have to be taken into account (5). A summary follows as Table 1.

Table 1. The educational system

Structure	Process	Outcome
Objectives	Meetings	Knowledge
Plans	Communication	Skills
Organisation	Group processes	Attitudes
Economy		Social effects
Trainers		Patient health
Trainees		

The evaluation committee had to decide on which parts of the educational programme to concentrate. All parts of the specialty training could not be covered, so the committee decided to use most of the resources on the process and particularly on the group work. This decision was in agreement with the aims of the evaluation. The structure, the process and the outcome cannot be understood as three separate parts. For example, if a lot of effort has been put into planning, the chances for success are greater than if you have to improvise. So even if we concentrated on studying the process, we also collected a lot of data about the structure and the outcome.

The next step in the planning process was to decide on what level the evaluation should be conducted. Evaluation can be carried out on four different levels; the individual, the group, the organization (the doctor's own practice) and society (the populations's health).

For different reasons the evaluation committee decided to limit the evaluation to <u>opinion</u> both at <u>individual</u> and <u>group</u> level. Evaluation of knowledge, behaviour or patient outcome would have required investigations before the doctors started their specialty training. Such studies are time-consuming and very difficult to carry out. Even if the doctors had improved their practice behaviour or changed attitudes after five years of training, the changes could not necessarily be attributed to the specialty training.

Two evaluation studies

The evaluation group published six reports and three articles during the two and a half years it was active. Summaries of two of the reports will be presented in this article.

The first intended to provide information for the purpose of adjusting the educational process if necessary. It was decided that methods designed to estimate the extent to which the participants' expectations were met could provide the information necessary for decisions to be made about the educational process (6).

After three months of group meetings (April 1986), the trainees were requested to make a list of up to 10 features they expected to find in such a programme. They were then asked to list the five most significant of these in order of importance, and then rate them on a five point scale according to the extent to which their expectations were met.

The ratings of the five selected features from all groups were compiled, analysed and categorized and the four most frequently mentioned by all groups were selected for further analysis. The four most frequently mentioned features were:

1. Increased comprehension of the characteristics and practice of general medicine (29 groups)

2. Good group collaboration (29 groups)

3. Facilitating the acquisition of medical knowledge (27 groups)

4. Evaluation of clinical problems and patient management (29 groups)

Eighteen months later (November 1987) a follow-up study was conducted. In between the groups had received feedback from the evaluation group. The purpose was to find out if the groups rated the features higher after having received feedback on their first ratings. The results are summarized in Table 2 below.

Table 2. The mean score of the groups' common ratings as to what extent the group has fulfilled the expectation of the feature in May 1986 and in November 1987

Features	Mean score	
	1986	1987
1. Increased comprehension of characteristics and practice of general medicine (29 groups)	3,8	4,1
2. Good group collaboration (29 groups)	4,1	4,5
3. Facilitating the acquisition of medical knowledge (27 groups)	3,6	3,7
4. Evaluation of clinical problems and patient management (29 groups)	3,5	3,6

The differences between the mean scores in 1986 and 1987 were not significant. Achievement of features 1 and 2 scored higher on both occasions than features 3 and 4.

Achievement of features 1 and 2 are general and could certainly be fulfilled without a formal teaching programme, simply by arranging informal meetings. Features 3 and 4, however, are different. They focused on the acquisition of knowledge and evaluation of daily encounters with patients, and corresponded to the two types of meetings in the tutor based part of the educational programme. Why their expectations were not fully met with respect to these features could be due to the fact that feature 2 (good group collaboration) was nearly fully met. The group members may have been too polite and so did not criticise each other and were therefore not really challenged on how they performed in the doctor-patient relationship.

The second study was based on written reports from the groups. In May 1987 the groups were asked to use half of a meeting to discuss their positive and negative experiences in regard to the training programme. They were also encouraged to suggest improvements to the programme. One of the trainees in the group was appointed to prepare a written report based on the discussion in the group concerned.

Thirty two of 38 groups responded by returning a written report. We found five common experiences.

1. The groups in sparsely populated regions had some practical and economical problems (one of the members in the group in Bodø had to leave home at 0430 in the morning and he returned home at 0700 in the evening. He travelled by car and plane. The costs were up to £1400 a year).

2. There was some overlap between the educational programme of the groups and the curriculum of the theoretical courses.

3. The groups followed the instructions of the Educational Handbook.

4. There was good group collaboration.

5. They developed increased understanding of the ideology and identity of general practice.

From our point of view, the most interesting reported experience was number 5. The trainees felt that participating in the group had given them increased understanding of the ideology and identity of general practice. Some groups reported that they valued this higher than being taught exact medical knowledge, for example: 'participating in the educational group has given us the opportunity to discuss the differences between general practice and the other specialties'; 'most of the trainees in the group had been working in general practice for more than five years without reflecting on the ideological basis for our work'. 'sharing experiences with colleagues in a friendly and open atmosphere has given us a common platform and thus increased our vocational self-confidence'.

Many general practitioners felt that the knowledge they had acquired in medical school was often irrelevant in their daily encounter with patients. It had become clear to them that a gap existed between the curriculum in the undergraduate study and the patients' demands and expectations. The specialty training has obviously aided in filling this gap.

This evaluation also disclosed that it could be expensive for doctors in rural areas to participate in the programme. To meet this problem the NMA has raised a fund so that expenses exceeding £1000 per year are reimbursed by NMA.

Conclusion

The specialty training for general practitioners in Norway was evaluated during a period of two years (1987-1989). The aims of the evaluation were: (1) to stimulate the educational groups to improve their way of working, and (2) to inform the specialty committee continuously so they could improve the training if necessary.

To fulfil these aims the evaluation committee needed an in-depth understanding of the educational processes. It was also necessary to maintain an open communication both with the specialty committee and the trainees. The evaluation committee therefore decided to use mainly qualitative methods.

The evaluation provided us with valuable information about the educational processes, and our good relationship with the specialty committee helped us to implement the results quickly. This was more important to us than carrying out a 'more scientific' evaluation using a rigorous methodological design in order to meet the demands of an objective evaluation.

References

1. Westin, S Utdanningshandbok for almenpraktikere (Educational Handbook for General Practitioners). Oslo, Gyldendal Norsk Forlag i samarbeid med Den norske laegeforening, 1986. English summary.

2. Harden, R M (1986) Approaches to research in medical education. Medical Education 20, 522-531.

3. Evans, E et al Does a mailed continuing education program improve physician performance? JAMA 1986; 255: 501-04.

4. Terpstra, D E Relationship between methodological rigor and reported outcomes in organization development evaluation research. Journal of Applied Psychology 1981; 66: 541-43.

5. Franke-Wikberg, S, Lundgren, U P Att vardera utbildning. Del 1. En introduktion til pedagogisk utvardering, Stockholm: Wahlstrom & Widstrand, 1982.

6. Rosinski, E F and Hill, P McN (1986) Student expectations and personal perceptions as an approach to course evaluation. Medical Education 1986; 20: 228-233.

CONTINUOUS ASSESSMENT IN VOCATIONAL TRAINING FOR BRITISH GENERAL PRACTICE

Donald Irvine - United Kingdom

Throughout the world, entry to most branches of medicine now conditional on completion of a programme of graduate or vocational training. Increasingly, this is true of general practice as well as the specialties. The nature of the training, and the standards of competence and performance required, are largely determined by those bodies which award professional qualifications. In the UK the medical Royal Colleges and their joint higher training committees have this role.

Specialty examinations have well known strengths and weaknesses. Essentially they tend to provide a reliable national standard for the assessment of those aspects of performance - especially of technical knowledge and problem solving skills - which can best be made using written tests, clinical examinations, simulated patient management situations and so on. What they cannot do is to show how well a doctor in training actually performs with patients and clinical colleagues under normal working conditions over a period of time. This constraint applies particularly to the assessment of certain attitudinal characteristics of performance - such as, for example, availability, punctuality, reliability, kindliness and a willingness to listen to patients. Yet these and similar caring characteristics are just as important to the overall performance a doctor as technical knowledge and skill. Patients and young doctors certainly understand that. Fortunately, such characteristics can be assessed to some extent within training programmes; and these assessments can be used to improve the validity of certificated performance.

In Britain, vocational training for the hospital specialties and health comprises a clinical apprenticeship and supporting academic courses. The medical Royal Colleges strongly influence such training through their accreditation of hospital posts suitable for teaching and through their professional examinations. Senior trainees are placed in numbered hospital posts which are approved for the quality of the experience and educational facilities they provide. The consultant trainers supervising these posts, who normally have no training in educational method, are encouraged to give trainees informal feedback on progress. The completion of specialist training is thus dependent on service in the right posts for the right period of time, and passing the College membership or fellowship examinations at the appropriate stage. In-service assessment plays an informal and relatively minor part in the process.

It was against this background that the Royal College of General Practitioners (RCGP) introduced the first experimental schemes of vocational training for general practice some 20 years ago. The RCGP sought to modify the specialty apprenticeship model in two important ways. First, it set out to enhance the value and consistency of the learning experience in general practice training posts, by ensuring as far as possible that trainers would be trained in educational method and would have their performance as clinicians and teachers regularly assessed. Secondly, the College urged the development of structured methods for the formative assessment of trainees with the object of fostering learning, encouraging trainees to monitor their own professional development, and in time moving towards a position where continuous assessment in training could weigh substantially in certificating competence and performance.

The development of these two approaches to continuous assessment in UK general practice are outlined in this paper. First, however, they need to be placed in the context of vocational training.

Responsibility for assessment

Three national professional bodies influence the standards of training for UK general practice. Vocational training and continuing medical education for all specialties are provided by the regional postgraduate organisations which bring the universities and NHS hospitals and general practices together in partnership. The Joint Committee on Postgraduate Training for General Practice (JCPT) sets and monitors national standards for training. Joint Committee certification is based on the aggregate of simple, subjective statements which trainers in general practice and hospital posts sign to indicate the satisfactory completion of each period of training.

The RCGP exerts an equally powerful influence on the content and objectives of training through its membership examination. The MRCGP examination is a voluntary exit qualification consisting of three written papers (an MCQ, a modified essay question paper, and a critical reading question paper) and two structured oral interviews. There are substantial regional variations in uptake and in the pass rate (1). In 1987/88 the overall pass rate was 74.7 per cent. In the same period over 95 per cent of trainees who sought JCPT certification achieved it, and so were eligible to become principals in the NHS. The Joint Committee, disturbed by the wide difference between its own and the MRCGP pass rates, is now encouraging the development of more objective methods for use in the continuous assessment of trainees.

The General Medical Council, which is the UK licensing body regulating basic medical education and coordinating all stages of medical education, will further influence standards of vocational training in all specialties when, in January 1991, it will indicate in the medical register those doctors who have been trained in a particular specialty including general practice.

Lastly, the regional postgraduate organisations are responsible for trainer and trainee assessment in training. The nature of this may be illustrated through the author's experience in the Northern region of England. It must be emphasised, however, that here again there are substantial regional variations.

Continuous assessment in the Northern Region

The Northern region has a population of just over 3 million people served by 1700 general practitioners. There are some 260 trainee general practitioners in general practice or junior hospital posts at any one time. Reflecting national policy, continuous assessment in the region involves both trainers and trainees.

1. Trainer assessment

The UK system for selecting trainers is operated by the JCPT and regional postgraduate organisations jointly. The JCPT publishes national guidelines for choosing trainers which should be reflected in regional criteria and standards. The Joint Committee uses its right to accredit training schemes and programmes as the means for keeping the regional trainer selection procedures under regular review. It seeks information about the performance of trainers and training practices, and it verifies this information by carrying out its own regular organisational audits of the postgraduate organizations; these audits include visits to randomly chosen practices.

In the early years both national and regional criteria emphasized the structural features of a practice such as the standard of the practice premises or the provision of a practice library. More recently the emphasis has been on the process of care and on the teaching provided. There are, for instance, explicit standards for clinical record keeping and for time earmarked for teaching in the practice; and there are implicit standards for access to care and for such clinical activities as prescribing and the management of chronic illness.

In the Northern Region trainer selection has been taken a stage further by the adoption of a contract for teaching services (2). To achieve this each practice and the regional postgraduate organization agree certain standards in advance on which selection will depend and against which subsequent performance will be assessed, and contracts renewed.

Amongst these standards, the contract specifies that a training practice will ensure that trainees acquire certain basic clinical and organizational skills which are considered to be essential for good medical practice. The skills are those required for the consultation, prescribing, clinical record keeping, performance assessment and practice management including teamwork.

Clearly if trainees are to learn these skills and to have their performance of them properly assessed, the partners of a training practice have first to establish their own standards and measures of performance. The more a practice makes such standards explicit for its own purposes, the easier it becomes to assess trainee performance because there is a defined context.

2. Assessing the practice

The main methods for assessing performance in British general practice are summarized below.

Practice inspections are invariably structured and are based on external review. The best known method is 'What Sort of Doctor?' (WSOD) introduced by the RCGP (3), in which four areas indicative of a doctor's performance are assessed, namely, professional values, accessibility, clinical competence and the ability to communicate. Assessment visits usually last for half a day, are carried out by a team of three experienced visitors and are repeated at three yearly intervals for the purpose of renewing the teaching service contract.

Practice activity analysis uses the potentially wide-ranging practice data on the process of care to examine patterns of, for example, prescribing, hospital referral, the use of laboratory and radiology services and other activities.

Case analysis involves the examination of randomly drawn patient records or it may be used for the monitoring of significant events such as unexpected deaths or cases where avoidable problems have arisen.

Clinical standards and algorithms may be used as 'tracers' of care to provide another window on assessment in general practice. For example, most Northern region trainers have just taken part in a regional study of standards and performance in which they constructed working clinical standards for five common conditions in childhood.

Surveys of patient satisfaction and patient outcome can reveal yet another aspect of performance. Trainees in the region also provide consumer feedback on trainer performance. They do this through their own surveys, and by completing a rating scale circulated confidentially by the postgraduate organisation.

3. Trainee assessment

The parallel approach to trainer assessment focuses on the trainee. In the Northern region the principal instrument is a rating scale designed to assess the performance of trainees in post. This has been complemented recently by MCQ, and OSCE (4), which have been organised regionally to provide trainees with further feedback on the state of their knowledge, skills and attitudes.

(i) New Manchester rating scale

When vocational training began the Region was one of three used to pilot a progressive rating scale developed by the late Professor Patrick Byrne of Manchester University (5). The Manchester Rating Scale, as it was known, consisted of a series of statements which derived from the job description of the general practitioner published in 1972 by the RCGP (6). This scale was used regularly in the Region in both the general practice and hospital components of vocational training for summative assessment.

Professor David Metcalfe has recently revised the Manchester Scale (7). The New Manchester Rating Scale is a more substantial document. Many Northern region trainers found it daunting to start with, but with local modification it is coming to be seen as the best instrument for continuous assessment currently available.

(ii) Content of scales

The New Manchester scales were constructed by a group of experienced general practitioner teachers. The first 15 of the 24 scales are devoted to rating the trainee's behaviour in every component activity of ordinary doctor-patient contact. Others cover emergency care, referrals to hospitals and aspects of the trainee's personal and professional development.

Each main scale consists of two statements which describe, on the left, the most undesirable behaviour that might be observed, and on the right, the most desirable. Raters are asked to indicate a trainee's current competence on a 10 point scale. The main scales are supplemented by very useful sub scales which develop particular aspects of the behaviours described in the main scale.

The trainer has several sources of information available when making assessments. These include video tapes of the consultation, the direct observation of consultations, record-based data indicating care given and significant events identified through monitoring, feedback from other members of the practice team, results of audits and simple observation and discussion.

(iii) The scales in action

During a six month period of attachment, the rating scales are normally used three times, at two monthly intervals. Because they are comprehensive, it is highly desirable to extend the exercise to more than one sitting. Some trainers use the scales privately to assess the trainee's progress. Others prefer to make the assessment jointly with the trainee, so to enhance the learning opportunities of the occasion. Yet others encourage self-assessment by the trainee first, using the scales; differences between the trainee and trainer assessments can then be fully discussed.

(iv) Experience with the scales

The scales are valuable in several respects. They act as a checklist or mini-curriculum. They help trainees to identify their strong points at an early stage, and so enable them to use their time and experience effectively by concentrating on weaker areas. They assist both trainer and trainee in recording progress. Operational weak points at present include inadequate hand-over arrangements when the trainee moves from one post to another.

4. Northern Region accreditation

The postgraduate organisation offers elective accreditation to trainees on the attainment of a satisfactory standard of performance in both the MRCGP examination and continuous assessment. These two approaches to assessment, although they overlap in what they measure to a considerable extent, are nevertheless concerned with somewhat different aspects of a doctor's competence and performance.

Experience to date indicates remarkably close results with both methods. However, there are outliers who have done well in the examination but whose performance at work has been sub-optimal, or vice versa. The fact that there are such outliers supports the argument for an accreditation which embodies both continuous assessment and an end-point national examination rather than rely on one or the other, for the two complement each other by measuring somewhat different aspects of performance.

In time it is hoped that this balanced approach will be adopted by the Joint Committee as the way forward with trainee certification on a national basis.

References

1. Royal College of General Practitioners. Annual Report. London: RCGP, 1989.

2. Northern Region education committee for general practice, The selection of trainers in general practice. Newcastle Upon Tyne; Northern Region Postgraduate Institute for Medicine, 1989.

3. Royal College of General Practitioners. What sort of doctor? Report from general practice 23. London: RCGP, 1985.

4. Jewell, D. Learning through examinations: use of an objective, structured clinical examination as a teaching method in general practice. Journal of the Royal College of General Practitioners 38 506-8.

5. Freeman J. and Byrne P A. The assessment of postgraduate training in general practice. Guildford: University of Surrey Society for Research into Higher Education, 1976.

6. Royal College of General Practitioners. The future general practitioner: Learning and teaching. London: British Medical Journal, 1972.

7. Metcalfe D H H et al. Rating scales for vocational training in general practice 1988, Occasional paper 40, London: RCGP, 1988.

ASSESSMENT IN ACTION

Professor David Metcalfe - United Kingdom

1. Assessment is a professional obligation:

To the trainee we owe formative assessment, to identify residual unmet learning needs; to the patients we owe summative assessment, to vouch for the competence of those into whose hands they will entrust their care; to society, which in one way or another pays for medical education in all its phases, we owe evaluation of our programmes, locally, regionally or nationally.

2. Assessment controls learning

When considering assessment it is important to understand the cultural environment in which it is to be carried out. Assessment is a polite word, usually, for 'examinations', even though there are a wider range of methods of assessment than there are of formal examinations. Examinations control learning. Not unreasonably, if further progress depends on passing the next exam, learners learn to pass that exam. If, for one reason or another that exam does not test the competencies to which the learning should have been directed, then those competences will not be learned. In the 60s the Royal College of Physicians had to redesign their Membership exam, and now the Royal College of Surgeons is doing the same thing.

In the UK at any rate, we belong to a 'pass and forget' culture: we take 10 subjects to the state examination GCSE at age 16, and dump seven of them; we take three, physics, chemistry and biology, to those at age 18, (the A level), and dump all three; we take anatomy, physiology and biochemistry for two years, and dump them when we get into 'real medicine' in the clinical course. Examinations then could be seen as giving the candidate, if he or she passes, permission to forget the learning acquired to sit them! In our society they have become the initiation ceremonies to allow us to enter adulthood, and when we have passed them we 'put away childish things'!

Because professional exams are such high hurdles, and are often extremely stressful experiences, they may leave traces long down the track of professional behaviour and development. For example, the theory on which final exams are based is that the consultation consists of taking a 'complete' history, doing a 'full' physical examination, making a diagnosis, and only then beginning to consider treatment. We are brainwashed into thinking that must be the proper way of doing things, and so, because for good reasons we don't do them, we must be inferior sorts of doctor! In the real world history and physical examination are selective hypothesis testing collections of data, and decisions about treatment will be early considerations in the transaction. Conversely mindless pursuit of a diagnosis before experimental treatment often harms and sometimes kills patients.

Assessment, therefore is not a freestanding event, but casts its shadow both ways, before and after, on learning and on professional development.

The excellent specialist must know all that there is to be known about his or her specialty; it doesn't matter how little he or she knows about any other specialty, (or even the world outside!). The specialist has to be narrow but deep. Those skills and knowledge are easy to test. The excellent GP is quite different: he or she has to know something about everything, all the specialties, behavioural science, epidemiology, and local conditions, even if not much. Moreover, he or she must be able to make linkages between these different areas, to form, for example a link between biochemistry and sociology when planning care for maturity onset diabetics. Width and powers of synthesis are much more difficult to test. The classical model of assessment in medicine comes from the teaching hospitals and is therefore specialist orientated.

Inappropriate assessment is characterised by over simplicity: this denies the richness of general practice and stultifies exploration. We have an obligation to assessment, but many opportunities to get it wrong, with serious results: we are playing for high stakes.

3. Validity and reliability:

Assessment seeks to acquire knowledge as a basis for action, whether at the formative (adjusted teaching), summative (qualification), or evaluative (programme change) level. The acquisition of knowledge as a basis for action is therefore research and must obey the rules of proper research. In particular it must be valid and reliable. Validity is the extent to which your measurement actually measures what you think it is measuring. Thus a test of knowledge has low validity if what you think you are measuring is competence.

Reliability is the extent to which your measurements are objectively true; hence the standard tests of test-retest and inter-observer agreement. In exams, reliability is essential for fairness.

In the 'hard' sciences, reliability is to do with generalizability and predictiveness, both qualities essential if the results are to be useful. In medicine, and general practice in particular, since all individuals are unique, generalizability and predictiveness are bound to be limited. It is amusing to see the behavioural sciences trying to attain scientific respectability by ever harder (more numerate) methodology in order to 'get into the physics lab', just as the physicists have gone out of the window into Heisenberg uncertainty! Spurious reliability is often bought at the expense of validity.

I have heard that there is something called Finagles Rule;

> 'The data that you have is not that which you want,
> The data that you want is not what you need,
> The data that you need is unavailable anyway!'

In assessment, reliability is fairness, while validity is meaningfulness. The multiple choice question (MCQ) is the best example of a method which is highly reliable, but largely invalid. Not only do we teach that 'there is no always and no never in medicine' and then, in the MCQ, ask if facts are True or False, but because of the difficulties of setting them we cannot ask lots of more important questions.

Case discussion, video analysis, or modified essay questions (MEQs) are all more valid, but a great deal of effort must go into making the marking reliable. Students distrust them, saying that the 'right' answers are 'only value judgements' (as if we didn't live most of our lives by value judgements). J K Galbraith said: 'The denigration of value judgements is one of the devices by which science maintains its misconceptions'.

Assessment must, if it is to be valid, first and always ask 'What is the research question: what are we trying to measure?'. Only when you have an answer to that can you decide whether the method of assessment chosen will answer it.

4. Assessment of learners:

In the assessment of individual learners, either formative or summative, the first question must be 'What are the aims of the learning programme?'. If there are no explicit aims, there can be no meaningful assessment. Anyone who failed such an assessment could justifiably say 'But that wasn't what I was trying to learn'.

If there are aims, at what level should they be expressed? They might be merely at the level of knowledge, which is easy to test, but which we know to be poorly related to competence. They might be in terms of knowledge, skills, and attitudes. It is harder to test these comprehensively, and it is important not just to go for the easy ones, putting more weight on tests of knowledge and observation of easily definable skills, for example those of physical examination, than on those of intellectual skills and attitudes. If the aims are expressed in terms of competence, then performance itself, rather than any surrogate for it, should be tested.

If the aim is stated in terms of competence, then observation of the activity in question would be most valid, but seldom practicable: not only would the assessors be spread all over the place, but their presence might skew the interaction. Conventionally such competence is 'laboratory tested' by observation under controlled conditions: the classical example would be the traditional clinical exam long case. The RCGP has always been accused, from inside as well as outside for lack of virility in not having a clinical examination in the MRCGP. But the clinical competence we are looking for in GPs is not the leisurely, inductive diagnostic exercise of the long case, who is bound to have some significant illness, classically with positive physical signs, because that's not we are trying to do. The essential competences are differentiating between minor illness that doesn't need to be gone into in depth, hearing the small but significant difference in the tale told by a regular attender which makes one 'change gear', and getting enough information confidently to exclude serious illness, and to do each of those things against pressure of time. To reproduce that in the examination 'laboratory' would be impossible. Denied of that ability we fall back on surrogates such as Modified Essay Questions and Objective Structured Clinical Examinations.

5. Assessment of programmes: evaluation:

This assessment is, by definition, an assessment of the extent to which the payers and the participants are getting value for money. It is important therefore to ask the questions in the right order:

> 'Is it effective?' (because if it is not, cost and acceptability are irrelevant); 'If it is effective, is it efficient?' (that is, does it achieve its objectives with minimal use of resources?); 'As long as it is effective and efficient, is it acceptable?' (that is do the participants enjoy it and like the way it helps them to learn?); 'If it's effective, efficient, and acceptable, is there equity?' (that is, is it equally available to all who are qualified to benefit from it and who wish to?).

If evaluation is to be valid, therefore, these are the questions it must ask, in that order. The first of these questions can only be answered if the aims of the programme are explicit, but the aims themselves are under review. When evaluating a programme the aims, given that they have been made explicit, must be subjected to the following enquiries:

- Are the aims related to the medical care needs of the people for whom these doctors are learning to care? (Are they, in other words, 'needs-derived'?).

- Are the aims resource sensitive? (Are they realistic in terms of the medical care system in which these doctors are going to work?).

- Are the aims up to date? (Do they relate to current patterns of illness, or those of the time at which the organisers went to medical school?).

- Do they reflect manpower realities, in terms of the number of doctors needed, the number of places available, and the gender-mix, both of doctor supply and patient preference? (For example, many women patients would prefer to see women doctors, but women doctors say, 'If I'd wanted to be a gynaecologist I'd have stayed in specialist medicine'. Is this addressed in training?).

If, and only if, the aims are appropriate in these ways can the next question be asked: 'Could the design of the programme achieve those aims?'. This is a difficult question to answer, because general practice is learned in complex ways. Nevertheless it is possible to form some judgement of course design. For example, since the competence aimed for is complex, the learning will be too: a single course of didactic lectures (or, for that matter all small group work) is unlikely to achieve it.

One way of coping, in evaluation, with the richness of the learning experience needed for general practice is to use Donabedian's categorisation into 'Structure', 'Process', and 'Outcome'.

Is the structure sufficient for the learning? Are there enough instructors with the right skills; is there suitable learning space; are there adequate supplies (audiovisual equipment, libraries etc); is the time properly divided between practical experience, instruction, and self-programmed time?

Is the process appropriate for the learning required? Is there the right mix of tutorial, group, didactic, and experiential learning opportunities; are the learning tasks in each properly designed; are they properly supervised; is there formative assessment?

What is the outcome? What are the results of summative assessment; what are the career achievements of the alumnae; what feedback from the learners is collected, and how is it used?

If the evaluation is to be valid, these are the questions that must be asked. They are all good questions to ask, but what sort of answers can we expect? Over and over again the word 'appropriate' crops up in plans for evaluation. Here reliability demands that criteria are set up and applied, and that those criteria are made explicit. Criteria will come from common sense and professional judgement, both of which are entirely justifiable bases for setting criteria. Once they are made explicit, comparing actual performance to them is not a matter of value judgements, and reliability can be achieved. A useful source of such criteria could be the learners themselves: after an introductory period they could debate their preferred ways of learning and their needs for time, space, support, and advice, with the training staff, and criteria could be agreed.

6. Summary:

Assessment is a professional obligation, to learners, the public, and those who pay for training and continuing education.

Assessment, however, exerts a powerful influence on the learning it tries to measure, and must be designed to reinforce that learning rather than distort it. Assessment is a form of research, and therefore must strive not only for validity and reliability, but also for a proper balance between them.

Validity can only be achieved when the aims of programmes are explicit; reliability depends on establishing the criteria by which structure, process, and outcome will be judged.

ASSESSMENT OF POSTGRADUATE MEDICAL EDUCATION - FUTURE DIRECTIONS

Marshall Marinker - United Kingdom

Introduction

Assessment is often represented as the guidance system of the educational process. However I will suggest that assessment may simply masquerade as the guidance system. Assessment can in fact become not only the guidance system, but also the map and the route.

Let me change the metaphor. The assessor is the monitor of our educational intentions, the friend, guide and protector of the innocents - that is to say the patients. But what kind of monitor is the assessor? Is he a friend and counsellor? Is he a policeman - the sort that helps old ladies across the road? There are, of course, other sorts of policemen - repressive, armed, secret and persecuting. Whose interest is the policeman protecting, and from whom?

Let me change my metaphor for a third time, in order to make my thesis clear. The assessments of medical education are a group of highly potent substances: small variations in the structure of these substances, and small variations in the dose, can transform a therapeutic benefit into a toxic disaster.

First, I am going to list three tasks of the general practitioner. Second, I shall suggest that there are four purposes of assessment. Then I will list three groups of factors which can be assessed. Finally, I will suggest four guidelines for future development.

Tasks of the general practitioners

Over the past 20 years there have been a number of attempts to describe and codify the tasks of the general practitioner in the overall provision of health care. Perhaps the most notable example was the publication almost two decades ago of The Future General Practitioner (RCGP 1972) which set out a blueprint for general practice training. Essentially three tasks were described.

The first task is the traditional biomedical one of clinical problem solving. The clinical task of the general practitioner contrasts markedly with that of the hospital based specialist. The task of the hospital specialist is to reduce uncertainty, to explore possibility and to marginalise error. The task of the general practitioner is to accept uncertainty, to explore probability and to marginalise danger. The general practitioner has to consider what uncertainties it is safe to accept when a child presents with acute pain in an ear obscured by wax, or when he considers what to do next for a middle-aged woman whose indigestion persists despite alkali mixtures and cimetidine. What probabilities does he need to explore when an adolescent girl loses weight, or when an octogenarian complains of giddiness on getting out of bed. What dangers must be marginalised when a child presents with high fever, or when a young woman presents with colicky abdominal pain?

The clinical competencies of general practice are derived from values which have lost ground in late 20th century medicine. What society values in our times is excellence in specialism, with an emphasis on technical skills, convergent thinking, rationality and the explicit.

Excellence in generalism has quite different characteristics. It is characterised by a superficial grasp of a very wide field of endeavour; problem solving is horizontal rather than vertical; thinking is as much divergent as convergent; the skills are not so much technical as interactive; there is room not only for the rational and the explicit, but also for the intuitive and the implicit. Do our educational assessments mirror the complexities and uncertainties of the general practitioner's biotechnical task?

The second task of the general practitioner extends the biomedical model to a biographical one. One of the central aims of vocational training for general practitioners in the UK, is that the doctor shall compose his diagnoses simultaneously in physical, psychological and social terms.

Although the phrase has an uncomfortably totalitarian ring, it enshrines an intention to value the patient as a unique individual, to understand the illness not only in biological terms but also in terms of the patient's feelings, social situation, health beliefs and much else.

The third task of the general practitioner relates to responsibility for the health of the practice population. Because of the structure of NHS general practice, each practice can define the exact population of persons who look to it for health care. This permits the practice to undertake health promotion tasks not only on a personal, but on a population basis.

The enthusiasm for all this prevention has tended to numb both scientific doubt and moral qualms about what is intended. Apart from childhood immunisation, many of these preventive measures are at least not sufficiently proven. Nor is the mandate to undertake this kind of activity altogether clear. Take the example of cervical cytology. Some studies reveal that as many as one third of the specimens examined are reported as being abnormal in some way. The cost, not simply the cost in medical resources but the cost in patient anxiety, has not been titrated against the hoped for good.

I have stressed the recent preoccupation with preventive medicine, to illustrate how powerful fashion has been in shaping postgraduate medical education for general practice. I have the feeling that assessment itself may now become the latest fashion to catch our fancy.

What are the purposes of assessment?

I want to suggest that there are four categories, under which we can consider the purposes of assessment. The first purpose I describe as absolutist; the second as contractual; the third as institutional, and the fourth as educational.

Let me begin with the absolutist. Here the intention is simply to enhance the quality of medical care. All sorts of questions are begged by this intention. What is the relationship between the educational process, its assessment, the subsequent performance of doctors and the quality of care which the patient will receive?

The absolutist position underscores all our efforts in medical education and its assessment. And yet every one of the links between what we teach and learn, how this is translated into performance at work, and how this performance influences the quality of health care, let alone the quality of health, remain leaps of faith, almost acts of worship. I am talking about our hopes for medical audit as teaching method, as management tool and as assessment. If this absolutist intention were the only one, or even the major one, then the profession could spend a large slice of the future in forging these links, in making them strong and durable. What saps our energy, and distracts our attention, are the contractual, the institutional and the educational intentions, which compete for our attention.

The second category of purposes can be described as contractual. A profession is characterised by a fiduciary compact between the professional and his client. This is served by the profession's intention, vigilantly to monitor its own standards. To this end bodies like the General Medical Council, the Royal Colleges, the Joint Committee for Postgraduate Training in General Practice, seek to assure the public that proper standards of training are maintained, and that the individual practitioners who emerge from the educational system are competent, and worthy of trust.

Professor Rudolph Klein believes that in modern Britain, the relationship between society and the professions (all of the professions not only medicine) is changing from one based on trust to one based on contract. He would be the first, however, to note that this shift from a relationship based on trust, to one based on contract, is not necessarily entirely in the interest of the patient or client.

The third category of purposes, I describe as institutional. By this I mean that the carrying out of assessment is a means of bolstering the power and authority of our professional institutions. Much of the power of the older Royal Colleges in the United Kingdom derived from their command of the higher diplomas in medical and specialist education.

In the Royal College of General Practitioners, for example, the examiners have reason to describe themselves not only as the guardians of the College's standards, but as the generators of the College's income. The examination produces members, and the members produce subscriptions. These facts create a massive disincentive to thinking about the examination, its relationship to training, its relationship to standards, its relationship to the meaning of membership of a professional body. Educational arguments can be snuffed out like feeble candle flames in the powerful winds of academic power politics.

The major postgraduate summative assessments, I have in mind the Membership and Fellowship examinations of the Royal Colleges, publicly signal professional competence in a particular field of medicine. Here, the assessment is no longer the handmaiden of medical education. Assessment, the examination, becomes the curriculum. If we are looking to the future of assessment, we must make sure that our assessments are more and more valid: closer and closer to our educational intentions, however complex, uncertain, intuitive and subtle these may be. In the quest for this validity, we must be prepared to sacrifice much reliability. Reliability in the end is concerned only with distributive justice, with being fair to the candidates in a competitive sense. In this pursuit of justice to the candidate, fairness to the intentions of the teaching, and above all fairness to the future professional needs of the men and women whom we are assessing, are dangerously and destructively ignored.

What can be assessed?

I want now to turn to what we can actually assess, and suggest that there are three groups of factors. The first group is associated with training. The second, with the quality of care which doctors give in practice. The third, often closely associated with the second but separate from it, is concerned with professional values.

The best of our effort goes into assessing the first group of factors - that concerned with training. At the most elementary level, we issue certificates of participation in courses and programmes of training. In essence our assessment of vocational training in general practice, has in the past been based on little more than evidence of satisfactory completion of a training programme.

In addition to compliance with attendance at courses, attempts are made to measure compliance with the intentions of training. The MRCGP examination is an example of this. But as I have already argued, it is the training which comes to serve the needs of the examination, and not the examination which comes to serve the needs of the training.

In the Manchester Rating Scale, there is an attempt to move away from the sort of measurements which one gets from an examination, to look at the way in which the teachers value the learners. Since I believe that vocational training in general practice should, first and foremost, be a series of personal apprenticeships, I approve of the Manchester Rating Scale. But my approval is conditional on the character, competence and excellence of the role models which we put before our trainees.

The second group of factors to be assessed are associated with the quality of care in practice. I am talking about medical audit. The possibility of rooting the whole of our Postgraduate Medical Education in the pursuit of medical audit is very attractive. After all, such a strategy will finally wed our educational intentions to the intentions of medical practice. We would learn what it is that we do, we would learn how to determine the goals of medical care, and how to achieve them.

But just like our professional examinations, our attempts at medical audit may have a most damaging and distorting effect both on medical education and on medical practice. For example, if our drive to measure performance is directed only by medical fashion, and by the seductive ease of measuring only the measurable, it will encourage a mechanistic and insensitive general practice which is at once compliant and unreflective.

You can see this already at work in the New Contract for general practitioners. This New Contract reflects the Royal College of General Practitioners' passionate preoccupation with the possibilities of preventive medicine - a passion which in the past decade has stilled both the scientific and the moral objections to many aspects of this enthusiasm.

The third category of factors which must be assessed, concerns professional values. Is it possible to assess the moral sensitivity of a doctor, his creativity, his willingness to look critically at his own performance, his sense of responsibility for the performance of his colleagues and so on? Exercises like the College's 'What Sort of Doctor?', the growing production in British general practice of Annual Reports which are written not only for the management of the practice, but also as a form of communication with the practice population, are examples of this.

It is impossible to avoid value judgements. But the evidence that such activities are going on, evidence that the activities are self-revealing and exploratory, not simply self-seeking and secretive, may be all that society requires, or should expect.

Future directions

Over the next decade, the need to think creatively about assessment may provide a new engine for the development of appropriate postgraduate education for general practice. Let me say that I believe that it will never be possible to reconcile satisfactorily the wish for validity in what we assess and how we assess it, and the wish for reliability. Perhaps we have to learn to accept in our educational process, the same sort of uncertainties that we have come to embrace in our approach to clinical medicine.

The future development of assessment in general practice may, however, help to resolve a major dilemma which we now face. Earlier I talked about Rudolph Klein's assertion that the relationship between society and the profession is now moving from one based on status and trust, to one based on contract. If our educational programmes, and our assessments, result in a morally and intellectually strengthened medical profession, one which could demonstrate a rigorous self-examination carried out without blame or punishment, a new fiduciary relationship between doctor and patient, between profession and state could be created.

If we are to achieve this new relationship, then our future thinking about assessment should be guided by four considerations. First, assessment must be developed as the servant and not as the master of the educational process. Second, it must move beyond the measurement of the retention of so-called facts and received wisdom, to an assessment of performance. Third, the performances which we decide to assess must not be solely determined by what we can reliably quantify. Fourth, we must devise techniques of assessment which look not only at training, but also at education.

Training simply prepares the learner to perform tasks already identified and described, by methods which have gained general approval. Training teaches us to solve puzzles, not to solve problems.

Education prepares us to solve problems. Indeed education prepares us to tackle problems the nature of which may not be known at the time that the education is taking place, and the solutions to which cannot be foreseen or even imagined by the teachers. The assessment of postgraduate medical education for general practitioners, must look not only at critical thinking,but also at creativity. It must be concerned not only with demonstrable competence, but with the capacity for personal growth. The challenge will be to bring to our thinking about assessment, something of the originality and audacity which general practice has already brought to medical teaching and learning.

References

RCGP (1972) The future general practitioner: learning and teaching. Royal College of General Practitioners and British Medical Journal, London.

RCGP (1985) What sort of doctor? Assessing quality in general practice. Report from general practice 23. Royal College of General Practitioners, London.

6. LEARNING FROM EACH OTHER

The UK-Nordic Medical Educational Trust

Peter Pritchard United Kingdom

Academic and cultural links between Nordic countries and UK date back to mediaeval times under the influence of King Canute (Knut) in the early 11th century. Visiting Dominican and Franciscan friars, some from Britain, started the 'studia generalia' in the 11th and 12th centuries, from which the universities evolved (Buttimer 1989). The incursions of the Vikings into Britain were perhaps less academic in their purpose, but they left a lasting cultural and genetic legacy.

We are now in the middle of a new renaissance of learning, not least in the field of general practice, that is affecting the whole of Europe. It is appropriate that once again we have an opportunity to share new ideas and knowledge. Focusing on cooperation between UK and Nordic countries, rather than the whole of Europe, has numerous advantages - of common culture, compatible health and educational systems, and Nordic people's fluency in English. However, this geographical focus can be interpreted as flexibly as future circumstances demand.

Though there have been sporadic visits between UK and Nordic countries in the past ten years or so, in my mind the turning point was the WONCA conference in London in 1986 which had stronger support by GPs from Nordic Countries than from Britain - to our shame. Professor Pertti Kekki of Helsinki University lit the fuse when he suggested that the WONCA conference would be a good opportunity to set up better cooperation between us. Accordingly a dinner was arranged in Covent Garden which attracted many of our most distinguished colleagues. Plans were laid for a UK-Nordic network to be set up, in order to exchange information, encourage mutual visits and set up a workshop. A questionnaire survey was undertaken to seek views on possible topics and format.

UK-Nordic Workshops.

The topics most favoured were: strategies for postgraduate training and education, methods of training, and evaluation of training. The level of consensus was high for the chosen topics. The first workshop was arranged to be held in London at the King's Fund College between 30th May and 3rd June 1990. There were 62 participants, and subsequent evaluation judged it to be a success. We were fortunate in receiving generous sponsorship both from Nordic and UK sources, without which the cost would have been a serious deterrent.

There was enthusiastic support for further workshops every two years, and Professor Paul Backer and the Danish College of General Practitioners have offered to host a workshop in Copenhagen in 1992. There was agreement that the topic should be related to general practice research. An educational topic was suggested for 1994 to continue the process started in London in 1990. Göteborg was suggested as a venue, with Professor Calle Bengtson as host.

The UK-Nordic Network

Potential participants were involved in the planning of the workshop and influenced the format, topics and venue. They contributed to the pre-circulated papers, and suggested the names of other people who might be interested. In this way a list of over 100 GPs was drawn up and the questionnaire and newsletters mailed to them. The number now is over 200, and is held on a computer database. A local coordinator of the network in each country has come forward, and their names are listed below. They will be linked electronically. The purposes will be to exchange information, to promote cooperation, to publicize the workshops and other events and to respond to requests for information. Help can be given to those who wish to visit each other's practices or to arrange fact-finding or educational visits. Members of the network will be expected to have something to contribute as well as being keen to learn.

There are many national and international institutions and agencies in Europe with related aims, but none to my knowledge that are specific to Northern Europe. There need be no serious clash of activities if the network resists the temptation to become an institution. By working at 'grass roots' level and in liaison with other organizations, it should be possible to reinforce cooperation and save duplication. This can be achieved by formal communication links and also through cross membership. Nearly all the members of the network are key people in other organizations.

UK-Nordic Medical Educational Trust

To secure the future of the network and other cooperative activities, a UN-Nordic Medical Educational Trust has been set up to act as a parent organization. Registration as a UK charity has been sought. Dr Godfrey Fowler is chairman of the trust, Dr Martin Lawrence the honorary treasurer and I am the honorary secretary.

We hope that the network and the trust will be flexible and responsive to new initiatives and ideas, so that it can be a channel for leadership at the same time as being 'demand-led' and participative. Anyone wishing to have more information is welcome to approach one of the coordinators listed overleaf.

Reference; Buttimer, A (1989). The wake of Erasmus. Saints, scholars and studia in mediaeval Norden. Lund University Press, S-221 00, Lund, Sweden.

COORDINATORS OF THE UK-NORDIC NETWORK

Denmark. Professor Paul Backer, Institut for Almen Medicin,
18 Juliane Maries Vej, DK-2100 Copenhagen Ø,
Denmark.
Tel 031 37 01 06, Fax 031 39 75 87.

Finland. Dr Outi Kupiainen, Lääkarinkatu 8C,
SF-00250, Helsinki, Finland.
Tel 90 470 2206, Fax 90 470 2900.

Iceland. Professor Johann Sigurdsson, Klettagata 17,
IS-220 Hafnarfjordur, Iceland.
Tel 01 652 600, Fax 01 65 36 00.

Norway. Bjørn Hoftvedt, Norwegian Medical Association,
Fjellveien 5, N-1324, Lysaker, Norway.
Tel 02 12 46 00, Fax 02 12 48 16.

Sweden. Dr Anna-Karin Furhoff, Karolinska Institutet,
Institutionem för allmänmedicin, Diagnosvägen 8 nb
S-141 54 Stockholm, Sweden.
Tel 08 774 94 74, Fǎx 08 711 44 48

United Kingdom. Dr Peter Pritchard, 31 Martin's Lane, Dorchester
on Thames, Wallingford, Oxfordshire, UK, OX10 7JF.
Tel 44 865 340 008, Fax 44 865 341 593.

Dr Godfrey Fowler, Department of Public Health and
Primary Care, Gibson Building, Radcliffe Infirmary,
Woodstock Road, Oxford UK, OX2 6HE.
Tel 44 865 319111 (& 319110), Fax 44 865 310 545.

7. HEALTH SERVICES AND GENERAL PRACTICE EDUCATION IN FIVE NORDIC COUNTRIES AND THE UNITED KINGDOM

Edited by Peter Pritchard.

Including, for each of the six countries:

Demography and health service organization,

Arrangements for general practice and primary health care,

Vocational (specialist) training of general practitioners, and

Continuing medical education of general practitioners.

Summary table

1. Denmark
2. Finland
3. Iceland
4. Norway
5. Sweden
6. United Kingdom
7. Figures and tables

The editor wishes to thank the Director of the Office of Health Economics for permission to reproduce material and tables from The Compendium of Health Statistics 7th edition (1989).

Table 7.1

Summary of data about five Nordic countries and UK

	Denmark	Finland	Iceland
Population (x 10^6)	5.1	4.9	0.25
Population density/km^2	119	15	2
Aged >65	15%	12.4%	10%
Aged >75	7%	5.5%	4.5%
%GDP on health	4.8%	7.4%	7.9%
£ on health pr person	349	770	900
% of health care on PHC	20%	32%	29%
% of health care on GP	7.8%	-	6%
No of doctors (total)	13,144	13,500	800
No of GPs	3,300	3,000	150
Patients pr GP	1,640:1	1,633:1	1,660:1
Employment	Self-employed	Salaried or self-employed	⅔ self-employed - ⅓ salaried
Staff (whole time equivalent)	<1/GP	Health centre	Health centre
Computerised	>5%	'some'	50%
Surgery consultations per day	26	20-25	15
Home visits	2.5	few	
Training			
Undergraduate - total (years)	7	6-6.5	6
- GP (weeks)	4	4-9	-
Pre-registration - hospital (months)	12	6	12
- GP (months)	6	5-12	-
Vocational training - total (years)	3.5	5	4.5
- GP (years)	150 hrs	2-3	2
GP as 'specialty'	no	1970	1970
GP training mandatory	yes	no	-
Continued education			
Reimbursed time per year	6 days	Paid by health centre	15 days
Problems	No locum	Limited budget	

Note - These figures are accurate to the best of our belief at the time of going to press. The editors wish to acknowledge the help they have had from authors of the papers and workshop participants (particularly Dr Anna Källqvist).

	Norway	Sweden	UK
Population (x 10^6)	4.2	8.5	57
Population density/km^2	11	21	234
Aged >65	16%	17%	15.6%
Aged >75	7%	7.3%	6.8%
%GDP on health	7%	9.1%	6.9%
£ on health pr person	900	1,050	450
% of health care on PHC	20%	23%	27.5%
% of health care on GP	6%		8%
No of doctors (total)	10,000	24,000	80,000
No of GPs	3,100	2,800	34,500
Patients pr GP	1,355:1	3,000:1	1,652:1
Employment	⅓ self-employed - ⅔ salaried	Salaried	Self-employed
Staff (whole time equivalent)	Health centre	2-3 pr GP Health centre	1.3 pr GP
Computerised	25-35%	'some'	50%
Surgery consultations per day	15-20	10-15	30-40
Home visits		few	3-4
Training			
Undergraduate - total (years)	-	5.5	5-6
- GP (weeks)	-	2-6	4
Pre-registration - hospital (months)	12	-	12
- GP (months)	6	-	-
Vocational training - total (years)	5	4.5	3
- GP (years)	2	2	1
GP as 'specialty'	1985	1981	1980
GP training mandatory	-	yes	yes
Continued education			
Reimbursed time per year	10 days salaried	Paid by health centre	5 days paid
Problems	No locum	Limited budget	

Additional sources: *Compendium of Health Statistics, 7th edition, 1989*, Office of Health Economics, London, and *Health Statistics in Nordic Countries in 1988*, Nomesko, Copenhagen, 1990.

Section 1
Denmark : Danmark

Demography and organization of health system

Dr Nicolaj Friderichsen

Demography

Population 5.1 million. Land area 43 000 km^2. Population density 119 per km^2. 326 800 are aged over 65 (13%), and 58 300 over 80 (2.3%). The rate of population growth is much lower than any other Nordic country and UK at less than 1 per 1000 population (1987).

Health service

In 1986, 5.7% of the gross national product was spent on health. In 1982 it was 6.2%. 7.8% of the health budget was spent on general practice (1988). 20% of the health budget was spent on primary health care (PHC) in 1985.

Health service organization

The Ministry of Health is responsible for the Danish health service and supervises it through the National Board of Health. The 15 counties are responsible for planning, finance and the day-to-day running of most health services. Local authorities are responsible for local services like district nursing, health visiting, school health and social welfare. Hospitals are mostly owned and run by the counties. A few are owned by patient unions. Two private hospitals have been opened - the first in November 1989. The Rigshospital in Copenhagen is owned by the State. All highly specialized functions are located in five of the larger Regional hospitals. There are no charges to patients for health or hospital care.

There are 13 144 doctors in Denmark of whom 3300 are GPs, 39 000 nurses and midwives, 5307 physiotherapists and 5164 dentists.

Organization of PHC

The general practitioner plays a central role in coordinating the care for a listed population. Danish GPs have a contract with the counties (NHS), which defines two categories from which patients may choose:

- Group I patients who must keep to their chosen GP for a year at a time, with the option to change GP each October. These patients need a GP referral to all specialists (except eye and ear) and to hospital. There are no charges to the patient. 96% of the population are in this category, and have free medical care.

- Group II patients can choose a different GP or specialist at will, but must pay part of the fee. 4% are in this category, and mostly live in big cities, where specialists are more concentrated.

Organization of general practice

There were 3300 GPs in Denmark in 1988 (1 GP to 1545 population). A large but unknown number of young doctors are heading for general practice. The vocational training scheme has a capacity of about 150 doctors per annum (see later). The number of GPs in a county is regulated so that each GP has an average of 1300 patients aged 16 and over. Children under 16 are not counted as patients, and are listed with their parents. This increases the numbers that the GP cares for by an average of 26% (22% children and 4% group II patients), resulting in a list of roughly 1640 patients.

The surgery premises are owned by the GP, who carries the cost of all staff and equipment, and also has to buy the goodwill of the practice on entry (estimated as up to 60% of the gross income of the practice averaged over the last 3 years). The GP is responsible for all organization and administration of the general practice. Health centres have not yet been introduced in Denmark, but they are a topic of some interest among politicians and health administrators.

The GP has to organize a 24 hour on-call service. Every practice has to be open from 0800 till 1600 Monday to Friday, plus one evening a week. Outside these hours, GPs can share the duties by a rota system, paid on a fee-for-service basis. Half the practices are single-handed, and the others are group practices of 2 to 7 GPs. Negotiations are now going on to extend the working day to 1800 and pay an hourly rate for out-of-hours duty.

Payment of the GP

The GP in Denmark is paid by capitation fee, a fee for each consultation, and fees for special services such as visits, laboratory tests and minor surgery. The capitation fee is 202 Kr (£18.3) per group I patient per annum. This is supposed to cover running costs, but seldom does so. The consultation payment is 41.35 Kr (£3.75).

The practice turnover per GP is about 900 000 kr (£81 000). Running costs average about 55% = 495 000 kr (£45 000), leaving 405 000 kr (£36 000) net before tax. But income tax is about 55%, so that leaves only 182 000 kr (£16 600) for the doctor. Living costs are higher in Denmark than in the UK.

The patient only pays for certain services such as certificates, health checks and special vaccinations. The billing system produces valuable statistics about practice 'output' which are used to control excessive use of services. The National Health service reimburses the cost of drugs and dressings for emergency use.

Consultations

During the day, a GP has on average 26 consultations and 2.5 home visits. After 1600 nearly all contacts are telephone calls or home visits. The length of the consultation averages 10 to 15 minutes. Urgent patients are seen at once or within 2 hours: less urgent appointments are often seen the same day or within a few days.

Staff and teamwork

In 1987 2662 GPs in 1517 surgeries had 3491 secretary/nurse/lab assistants (400 full-time: 3091 part-time). PHC is carried out jointly by the general practitioner and nursing staff employed by the local authority. The PHC team includes the district nurse, the health visitor, the school doctor and nurse and the school dentist. The GP takes care of the child immunization programme which is financed by the State. Meetings with the primary health care team are not included in the GP's contract, but regular telephone contact is maintained, and some practices have joint meetings with other team members. Most local authorities have a GP as consultant. Larger cities employ full-time community health doctors.

Family planning

This is mostly carried out by the GP, but in some larger towns there are clinics run by local authorities.

Alternative therapies

These are very popular in Denmark. Only chiropractors get reimbursement from the NHS. Figures for the extent of public use of alternative therapies are not available.

Private practice

There is virtually no private general practice in Denmark, apart from a few doctors who practice acupuncture and osteopathy.

Laboratory and X-ray services

Normally the GP takes the blood sample and does simple tests in the surgery. For more complex tests, either the patient or the blood is sent to the hospital laboratory. The patient does not pay. No GPs have X-ray equipment, but it is available on referral to hospital.

Computers

5% of practices have a computer, and the number is increasing rapidly. Some practices have a link with laboratories for receiving test results. No computer data goes outside the practice. Case notes belong to the GP.

Complaints

Patients can complain about a doctor or about treatment to the Ministry of Health. Complaints are rare and are seldom accepted as reasonable.

Personal comments

The author thinks it important that two thirds of the GP's income comes from consultation fees and one third from capitation in order to encourage the doctor to do as much for the patient as possible in the primary care setting, and only refer when the problem is beyond his or her capacity.

See organization chart overleaf.

Organization of health services - Denmark

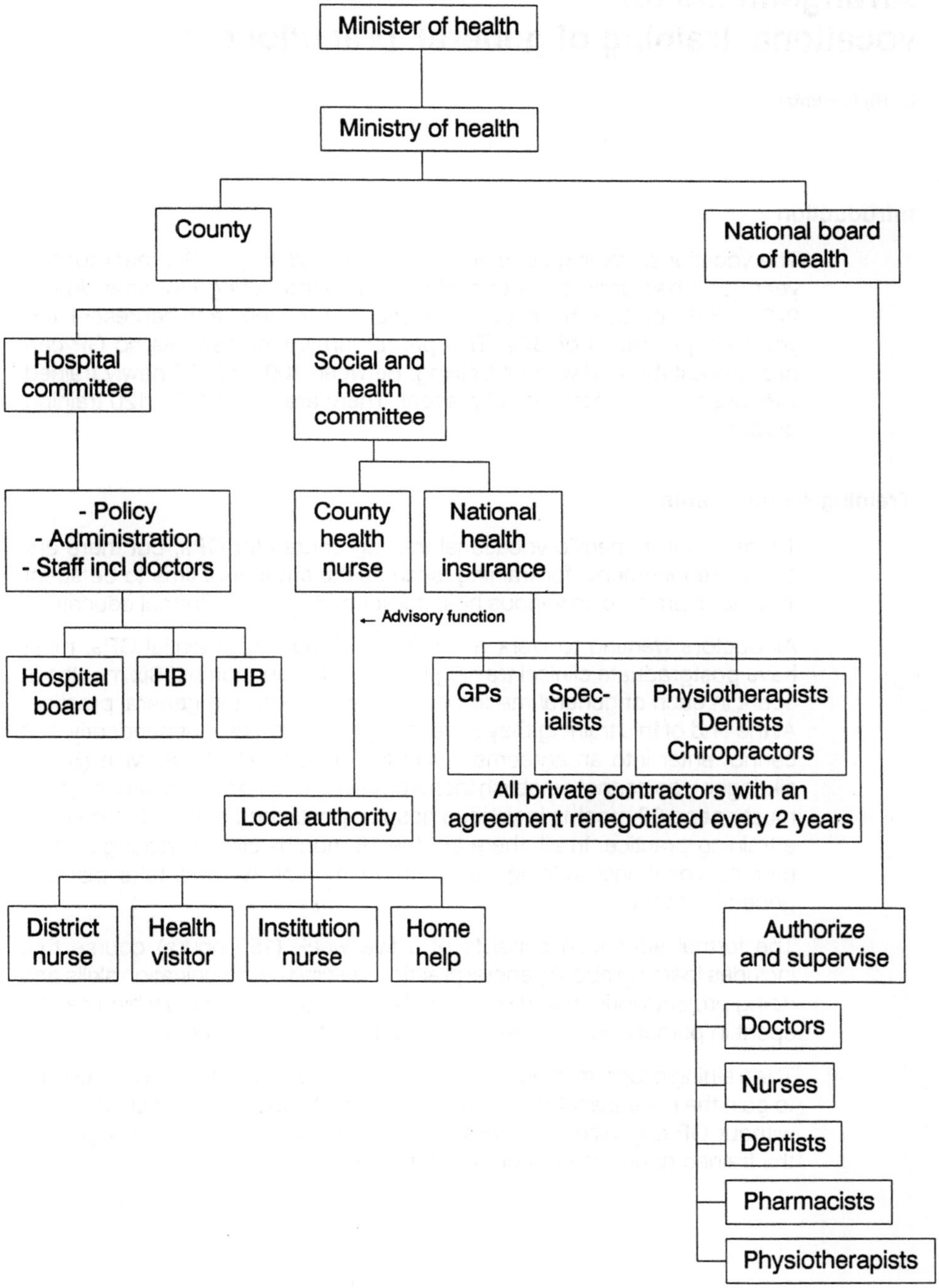

Arrangements for vocational training of general practitioners

Dr Niels Bentzen

Introduction

The vocational training scheme has been mandatory in Denmark for ten years and has undergone considerable change during that time. About 22% - 30% of GPs have been vocationally trained, and represent the younger generation of GPs. This proportion will increase as no GP can become established without training. Between 100 and 150 newly trained GPs are needed each year at present. There are about 100 - 120 training practices.

Training requirements

There is not a specific vocational training course for GPs, but there are certain requirements for training, such as the amount of time to be spent in general practice, in various hospital specialties and in formal education.

All doctors wanting to work as clinicians, including potential GPs, must have postgraduate clinical training lasting eighteen months. Six months is spent in each of general medicine, general surgery and general practice. At the end of this training they have the right to practice independently, but cannot enter into an agreement with the National Health Service (Sygesikringen), so cannot establish themselves as GPs. For this to happen, they must spend 30 months in various hospital posts, and at least 6 months in a training practice. In all, there are the 18 months clinical training and 42 months vocational training, of which 12 months have to take place in general practice.

The formal education consists of a five week (150 hours) course that includes learning about general practice, gaining communication skills and doing project work. In addition there is an optional 6 months which can be spent in primary health care units or university departments.

The training programme is not set out in detail, but each trainee is expected to gain the necessary knowledge, skills and attitudes through clinical work without GP-organized supervision. The training practice must supervise the trainee during the 6 months spent there.

Assessment

There is no formal assessment after clinical training, nor an examination at the end of the formal course. There is no reassessment of practicing GPs.

Selection of trainers

There is no prior assessment of trainers, except that they should have been in practice for 3 years and have at least 1000 patients on their list. New requirements about the facilities of the practice and the willingness to teach have been proposed by the Danish College of General Practitioners (DSAM) and the General Practitioners Association (PLO). Hopefully this voluntary code and self- selection process will root out the bad teaching practices and clarify the aims of the good ones.

University input

There is no formal university input into vocational training, but university teachers are closely involved with the formal education courses. They also run voluntary evening teaching, and courses for trainees and trainers. There are no specialist university degree courses in general practice. A number of courses for teachers have been arranged, but attendance is not mandatory.

The future

A future goal is to get general practice accepted as a full specialty in its own right. Before this can happen there must be firmer and better selection criteria for teaching practices. Another goal is to extend the vocational training time in general practice to 18 months, instead of 6 months as at present; so extending the total period of GP vocational training from 42 to 54 months, (after the compulsory basic 18 months of clinical training). The process is a slow one, with changes taking a decade, but we all hope that this goal will be reached before the year 2000.

Arrangements for continuing medical education of GPs

Dr Mogens Johansen

Introduction

All doctors in Denmark have an obligation to engage in continuing medical education (CME) in order to keep up to date with developments in their field. The Danish Medical Association (DMA) as well as the county medical associations have the responsibility to ensure that a number and variety of educational activities are available to all doctors, including GPs.

Administration of CME

The opportunities for CME for GPs in Denmark are plentiful. All GPs have a contract with the National Health Service (NHS) which means that our livelihood depends to a great extent on the number of registered patients, as well as the number of services rendered. The NHS allows for 6 days CME per annum, and GPs are reimbursed for loss of income. The course fees are paid by participants themselves, but these can be set against income tax. As a result, most GPs can undertake 6 days CME without financial loss. However, each GP only spends about 2.6 days on CME. Furthermore, only about one GP in three takes advantage of these arrangements. These figures only refer to courses requiring absence from work, so evening meetings, short symposia or weekend courses are not counted.

Varieties of CME

- Centrally organized CME

Centralized courses are arranged by a GP committee of the DMA. 18 - 20 residential courses are arranged each year with a duration of 2 to 5 days. About 24 to 100 GPs attend. The subjects include the updating of general medical knowledge and also topics in which GPs have not had formal education - for example psycho-therapy, crisis care, the diagnostic process, the doctor in society and home care of the elderly etc. Courses are also held in research and teaching. Suitable locations are chosen where modern educational technology is available such as role-play and video techniques.

- Locally organized CME

  The county medical associations also have a course committee responsible for CME for GPs, junior doctors and specialists. The activities vary, but are mostly short courses and evening sessions. The participants are 40% GPs, 60% junior doctors, but practically no specialists. The Danish Society for General Practice has previously arranged courses, but now mostly sets up individual instruction.

- Sponsored CME

  Pharmaceutical firms are very active in CME for GPs, mostly arranging short symposia and evening meetings of a high standard, held 2 or 3 times a month and addressed by hospital specialists. Attendance is often very good.

- Small-group CME

  About one third to half of all Danish GPs have organized themselves into so called '12-man groups'. These groups (of 8 - 14 GPs) live near to one another and may be involved in a duty rota. They meet 6 to 12 times a year without a formal programme, in order to exchange experiences from their practices, and sometimes to engage in medical audit. Some of these groups work extremely well and are strongly supportive of CME. They have also raised the level of understanding of the problems of general practice among those working in the field. Some GPs form discusssion or therapeutic groups, and Balint groups of 4 - 8 people, often with a qualified group leader, either a psychologist or a psychiatrist.

- Academic CME

  Finally, some CME takes place within the Institutes of General Practice in Copenhagen, Odense and Aarhus - particularly in the areas of research and teaching.

Personal views of the future

There have been major experiments and positive experiences in the field of CME in Denmark. Participating GPs seem ready to accept very innovative forms of education. A current topic is whether Danish GPs are getting enough CME, and the general feeling is that they are not. There is at present no obligatory CME nor formal re-accreditation.

Section 2
Finland : Suomi

Demography and organization of health system

Dr Marjukka Mäkelä

Demography

Population 4.9 million. Land area 338 145 km^2. Density 15 per km^2. Helsinki, the largest city, has a population of half a million. Northern Finland extends to the 70th parallel of latitude, further north than Iceland and level with the middle of Greenland, and is sparsely populated. Over 60% of the population lives in towns. 93% speak Finnish: 6% speak Swedish as their mother tongue. Population growth has been relatively slow, (3 per 1000 population in 1986). The population over 65 has grown by 7.4% in 1960 to 12.4% in 1984, and is expected to rise to 15% in the year 2000.

Health service

Since the introduction of the Community Health Care Act in 1972, health care planning has been systematic, with national five-year plans. National planning ensures the support of underdeveloped areas, such as rural primary health care (PHC), by allocation of resources.

7.4% of the gross national product is spent on health, and of the health budget, 32.4% is spent on health centres and 37.2% on PHC (including environmental and occupational health).

Health service organization

Local authorities are responsible for provision of health care services. The State provides between 29% and 66% (average 42%) of approved expenditure on PHC, depending on the financial status of the local commune (local government district). Smaller communes can join together to provide PHC. Communal hospital federations are responsible for central and regional hospitals.

Organization of PHC

The health centre is the unit through which all PHC services are provided for the population of a defined area, usually a minimum of about 10 000. There are 215 health centres in Finland employing over 50 000 people on a salaried basis. They provide promotive, preventive, curative and rehabilitative services. In addition they provide in-patient services having a total of 23 000 beds. The Communal Board of Health is the body responsible for the provision of services, and day-to-day administration is in the hands of a team consisting of the chief general practitioner (GP), the head nurse and the health centre manager. 3010 GPs (22% of all doctors) work in health centres (Jan 1989). There are 660 vacancies for health centre GPs.

Health centres

A health centre is an organization not just a building, as in UK. There may be several 'health stations' for providing PHC. They offer a wide range of services, including health education, maternal and child health, school health, dental care, laboratory, physiotherapy, X-rays, ambulances and minor surgery. The health centre wards provide acute medical care, day care, intensive rehabilitation and long-term care.

Health centre staff

A typical Finnish health centre, providing services for a population of 25 000 (including in-patients) would employ 140 people, as listed:

- 10 general practitioners
- 19 registered nurses
- 20 auxiliary nurses
- 12 public health nurses
- 8 dentists
- 3 laboratory technicians
- 1 X-ray technician
- 2 physiotherapists
- 30 other health professionals, including a psychologist, speech therapist, social worker, dental technicians, health centre aids, and 35 clerical and domestic staff.

Teamwork

There is a long tradition of teamwork in Finnish health centres. The core team consists of a general practitioner, a public health nurse and a health centre aid. The extended team includes the professionals listed above and teachers or patients' relatives as appropriate. Coordination of services and continuity of care work well with team responsibility for a small geographical area.

GP consultations

The time reserved for non-urgent appointments is 15-20 minutes. For acute problems, 10-15 minutes is typical. For preventive work, 20 minutes of medical time and 30-60 minutes of nurse time is reserved.

Waiting time

57% of urgent cases wait for less than an hour. Non-urgent cases wait an average of 12.6 days from booking an appointment (range 2 - 25 days).

Payment of GPs

Health centre GPs have, up to now, received a basic salary of 10 000 to 13 600 FIM per month (about £18 000 to £25 000 per annum). There are additional fees for out-of-hours work, certificates and special procedures. These total about 4000 FIM per month (about £7000 per annum).

Private practice

There is an increasing number of private health stations, mostly in large cities. 500 doctors work in private occupational health schemes and there are 750 private GPs. These account for 20% of visits to GPs. About half the cost of private health care is paid by the State. Occupational health care is subsidized also.

What patients pay

Patients do not pay to see a GP. Transport is subsidized for sums over 50 FIM (£7.70). Prescriptions are issued free. Patients pay half of the drug costs, except in the case of certain vital drugs for chronic conditions when the patient pays either nothing, or up to 10% of the cost. Patients pay 65 FIM (£10) per day for stay in hospital, and 50 FIM (£7.70) for an outpatient consultation.

Computerization

Some communes have established computerized systems for appointments and laboratory results only. Some have entire medical records on computer, with advanced network links with laboratories, hospitals and satellite health stations. However, most are in the stone age. Finance comes from local health boards. Access to patient data is normally confined to health care personnel. Data protection is built into computerized record systems. For research, a permit must be obtained from the communal Board of Health. The personal identification number used throughout the health and social services makes it possible to link data for research, once the official permit has been given.

Laboratories and X-rays

All health centres have laboratory and X-ray services in the building or nearby. The cost is covered by the health centre budget. 19 million laboratory tests were done at health centres and 1.8 million X-rays taken in 1987.

Other facilities

All health centres have space for minor operations. Some have theatres for deliveries and caesarean sections, or minor surgery such as haemorrhoidectomy or vein stripping.

Prevention and screening

The preventive services are mainly offered in health centres where mass screening and immunization campaigns are carried out. The exception is the two thirds of occupational preventive care which is privately delivered. The GP heads the preventive team, and she performs, for example, 20% of maternity care and 50% of well-baby checkups herself.

Complaints procedures

Complaints are mainly handled within the health centre organization. If necessary a patient advocate can be approached and complaints taken to the National Board of Health.

Alternative therapies

The National Board of Health controls the majority of alternative therapists. Their services are widely used - over 10% of the population uses at least one form of alternative therapy, even though there is no reimbursement of the cost.

Secondary care

In general, patients are referred to secondary care. There is, however, direct access to emergency departments, and patients can be referred by nurses or private practitioners.

Medical manpower

There is an increasing shortage of personnel in health care. 33% of posts for physiotherapists are vacant, and 17% of GP posts. There is also a shortage of health centrė nurses and aids. This is partly due to the increase of private medical facilities. Local variations are great.

Further reading

1. Kekki, P. (1986) National perspective: Finland. In Fry J and Hasler J (eds) Primary Health Care 2000. Churchill Livingstone, Edinburgh.
2. Ministry of Social Affairs & Health and National Board of Health (1987) Health care in Finland (2nd edn). Government Printing Centre, Helsinki.

Organization of health services - Finland

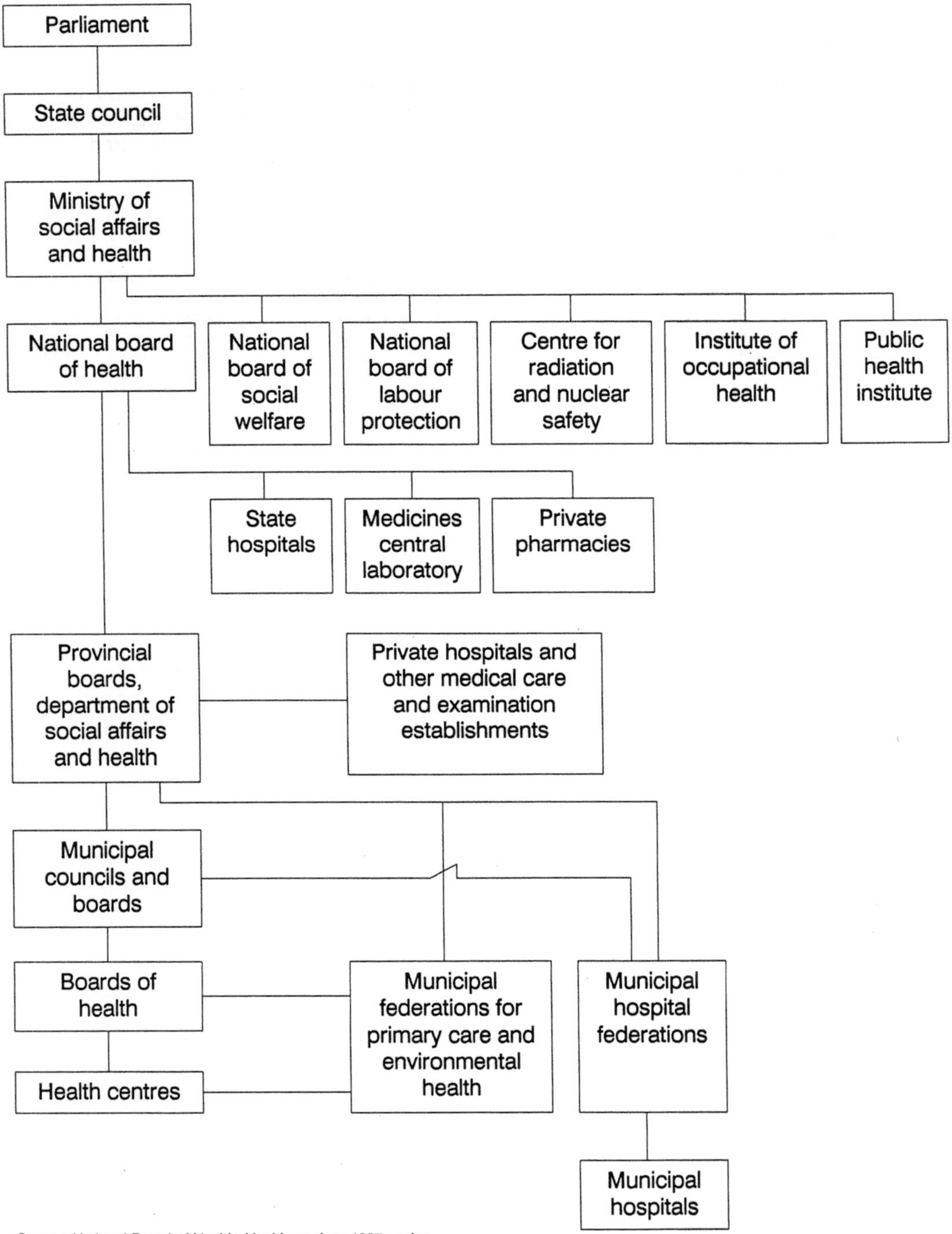

Source: National Board of Health: Health services 1987. series Health 1989:3:p.9. Government printing centre, Helsinki 1989.

Arrangements for vocational training of GPs

Dr Irma Virjo and Professor Mauri Isokoski

Extent of vocational training

Of the 13 511 doctors registered in Finland on 1 January 1989, 51% were vocationally trained: 1040 general practitioners (GPs) in Finland were specialists. The specialty of general practice has existed in Finland since 1970. About 20%-25% of GPs working in health centres were vocationally trained. Some GP-specialists work in other tasks in public health care and some in the private sector. On 1 March 1989 there were 1859 doctors undergoing training in all specialties. 270 (14%) of them were in training for general practice in the four universities which have this programme.

Responsibility for vocational training

The National Board of Health was responsible for vocational training of all specialties until August 1986, when most were transferred to the universities. Responsibility for general practice training was transferred two years later. Specialization in general practice is still possible under the old regulations until July 1991. The new training programmes for general practice, with defined objectives, were confirmed in 1988.

There are now chairs of general practice (and/or PHC) in four out of the five Finnish universities. The professors are responsible for the training programme, but were not initially resourced for this new function.

A prerequisite for vocational training is a degree in medicine (usually 5 to 6 years), followed by 6 months in hospital and 6 months in a health centre, or 1 year in general practice. The programme lasts 5 years and is outlined below.

Programme of vocational training

- General training (1 year consists of full time work in any medical post; then:
- Special training consisting of 2 to 3 years work in a health centre and 2 years in hospitals posts approved by the National Board of Health. These posts can be in different (but defined) branches of clinical medicine (for example four posts of at least 3 months each). The trainee can plan the programme, but it must be acceptable to the professor.

During these 5 years the trainee must participate in regular in-service training.

Formal education

The trainee must also participate in courses of training (120 hours), of which 20 hours is in administration. This education may be organized by the university or, for example, by the College of General Practitioners. All courses must be approved by the university and the trainee must negotiate the content of the programme with the professor. Small group work is used to some extent.

Required reading

There is a list of five textbooks, four by UK authors and one USA, and five journals from the past three years (one Scandinavian, two UK and two Finnish). General directives about primary health care must be studied.

Training methods

These vary in different universities, but to take the example of the University of Tampere, the principles of self-directed learning (Malcolm Knowles) are used. The trainee, together with the professor, makes a learning contract where the trainee is responsible for his or her learning. In seminars of 10 to 20 trainees, the GP's work is analysed, and the trainees must each identify their own learning needs and plan the programme accordingly. Not all universities follow this approach, and in some the more traditional teacher-centred methods are in use.

Work experience

The trainee must work as a GP in approved posts under the guidance of a more experienced doctor. This involves discussions and the possibility to consult when needed. Some GP trainers use indirect supervision in which the trainee describes patient cases. Video is rarely used in supervision.

Assessment

At the end of vocational training there is an obligatory national examination consisting of essay questions. Once the trainee has followed the approved training modules and passed the examination, he or she may apply to the National Board of Health for registration as a specialist in general practice. There is no re-assessment at present.

Selection of trainers

Under the old regulations it was not necessary to appoint a trainer or supervisor. Now all hospital and health centre posts are accepted for training, and there is no selection of trainers. There are problems of shortage of GPs experienced in training and lack of staff at universities. The University of Helsinki is arranging education courses for trainers. Eventually, it is hoped that all trainers will themselves have been trained as teachers.

Integrated training

In some areas, for example Helsinki, one application will ensure the whole range of posts and training needed: in others the trainee must apply for each post separately. Integrated training is a goal for the future.

Future goals

The organization of vocational training is being built up and is still developing. One goal is that after 1 August 1991 only certain health centre and hospital posts will be approved for GP training. The following criteria are used for health centres:

- there is a post for a GP trainee.
- there is a specialist in general practice who is suitable and willing to be a trainer, who has participated in teacher training and has time reserved for the training task.
- the range of services offered is wide enough.
- there is organized in-service training of at least two hours a week.
- there is a library with at least the required literature.
- the trainee is able to participate in the more formal educational courses.

The eventual goal is that all GPs employed in health centres will have successfully undertaken a vocational training programme of high quality to fit them for their very important, but demanding life work.

Arrangements for continuing medical education of GPs

Dr Katia Käyhkö

Introduction

Arrangements for GP continuing medical education (CME) in Finland vary in the five university centres. In addition, the Finnish Medical Association arranges annually a one-week continuing education conference in Helsinki. This conference covers most specialties and thus covers many topics. Usually this conference (Medicine-90) includes one or two day-long courses which are intended for GPs. The Medical Scientific Association 'Duodecim' also arranges annual regional conferences in the cities of Tampere, Kuopio, Oulu and Turku. These conferences resemble the main annual events in Helsinki in all respects but duration which is three days.

All continuing educational events are open to all doctors in Finland and all the courses of the Department of General Practice and Primary Health Care are likewise open to both private doctors as well as health centre doctors. It can be assumed that almost every GP attends some kind of continuing education annually. The courses arranged by the Department of General Practice and Primary Health Care of the University of Helsinki are attended every year by approximately 300-350 doctors. The programme of the University of Helsinki is the oldest and most comprehensive CME program for GPs, and this will be described here in detail.

Clinical CME

CME courses on clinical topics have been in operation since 1979. They are open to GPs and other health care personnel, depending on the topic. There are 9-10 topics covered and each course lasts five days. The topics include paediatrics, surgery, geriatrics, gynaecology and maternity care. The teachers are from the University specialist departments. The number of participants is limited to 30. The courses are held at a picturesque educational centre 100 km north of Helsinki.

The course and residential fees (amounting to 2500 FIM, about £370) are paid by the health centre which employs the GP.

Non-clinical topics

In addition to the clinical courses, the Helsinki University department of General Practice and Primary Health Care arranges other courses for GPs, using its own teaching staff. The topics include research methodology in Primary Health Care (PHC), quality assurance and physiotherapy. These courses are modular (ie in several parts, with several months in between). They are aimed at the PHC team, and members of more than one professional group are required to attend. There is much group work, and project work done between course modules. The aim is for team members to 'learn by doing' in a multi-disciplinary group setting.

Trainer courses

Annual courses for GP trainers have been in operation in Helsinki since 1985. These are of one week's duration, and focus on learning theory, individual or small-group teaching, and observation and feedback. Teachers of GPs and of medical students attend, and the courses have been very popular.

Teaching projects in health centres

The main focus of CME in the department has, however, been on collaborative teaching projects in health centres. These are based on integrated problem-orientated, competency based, multidisciplinary education. These projects are arranged at the request of health centres. They have been seen as a point of entry into development activities in the health centre. Health centre personnel are encouraged to identify their own problems and educational needs, in keeping with the principles of a quality assurance project. They then collect and analyse data (under the guidance of the department), implement changes and measure outcomes. These projects are financed from the education and development budgets of the health centres.

Role of pharmaceutical companies

The continuing education arranged and sponsored by pharmaceutical firms in Finland is extensive in numbers of events, but it is sporadic and primarily serves the firms' promotion and marketing interests. The topics are clinical and usually the lecturer is a hospital specialist. These educational events last from a couple of hours to one day.

Evaluation of CME

Extensive research in several health centres in Finland[1,2] has shown the need for specific and supervised training in collaboration between the various professional groups. The educational projects described have enhanced teamwork and the provision of comprehensive and effective care.[3]

All the CME described above has been popular with PHC personnel. The integrated problem-orientated model described above is seen as the most effective vehicle for CME in the setting of PHC in Finland, and is also in line with World Health Organization strategies for PHC development.

References

1. Kekki, P. Assessing the Management Effectiveness in Health Centres. An example of the use of a tracer activity in the evaluation of primary health care. World Health Forum, in press.
2. Kekki, P, Sihvonen, M. Health Centre Efficiency. First results of an organizational analysis of four Finnish health centres. Scand J Prim Health Care 1989; 7: 143-7.
3. Kekki, P. Training for primary health care. World Health Forum, in press.

Section 3
Iceland : Island

Demography and organization of health system

Dr Jóhann A Sigurdsson

Demography

The country is an island with an area of 103 000 km^2, placed in the north Atlantic. Its northernmost part reaches the Arctic Circle, and Reykjavik, the capital town of Iceland, is on the same latitude as Umeå in Sweden, Trondheim in Norway and Vaasa in Finland. The total population is only a quarter of a million and of those 60% live in the capital town and its surroundings.

Health spending

The Icelanders spend 7.9% (1985) of their gross national product (GNP) on health services. About 70% of this sum goes to hospitals and sanatoria, 6% to general practice and primary health care, 7% to specialized services outside hospitals, 6% to dental services and 10% goes on pharmaceutical services.

Organization and administration of health service

The health service is administered by the Ministry of Health and Social Security, which was established in 1970. It is headed by the government and the cabinet minister. The formal administration of health care takes place in three levels, a) the state, b) the regional authorities and c) local boards.

As the population is small, the state plays a central role dealing with construction and establishments of hospitals and health centres, and legislation. Medical supervision is mainly the responsibility of the Directorate of Public Health.

The country is divided into eight regions (municipalities). Each region has its own health council. One of the GPs in the area is appointed to be regional chief medical officer, heading the council. At least one hospital and many health centres are placed in every region. The main objects of the councils are to plan, recommend and prioritize the main tasks of the health service in the area and to coordinate the activities of the health care institutions.

Hospitals

Because of the great number of small villages and towns around the country, some of which are isolated, there are many small hospitals with 20-60 beds. The hospitals are divided into categories according to their capacities. The total number of beds (in 1988) was 4340 which equals 17.5 beds/1000 inhabitants. In addition, there were 1700 special homes and apartments for old people in various categories.

Health centres

In 1973, the Icelandic Parliament decided to establish new health centres all around the country. This enormous project is almost completed with a total number of 79 health centres. This favourable evolution has been somewhat slower in Reykjavik than expected in the beginning, with only five health centres out of a total of 14 planned in that area.

The health centres are divided into three categories: H2, where there are at least two GPs with other personnel (35 centres in all); H1, where there is only one GP with other personnel (17 in all); and H (27 in all), where there is only a nurse or a midwife with regular visits by the nearest GP. The catchment area of each health centre is from 1000 to 15 000 inhabitants.

Staff

In Iceland there are about 7000 persons employed in the health service (2.8% of all inhabitants) and of these, 500 (7%) are working in primary health care. The total number of doctors in Iceland is 800 (one per 315 inhabitants). There are 150 GPs (19% of all doctors) which means one GP per 1660 inhabitants. The number of GPs with special education in family medicine is increasing and is now up to 67 doctors (45% of all GPs). There are still very few women working as GPs, only eight at the moment and of those four have postgraduate education in family medicine. 25 GPs (17%) are running their own private practices.

How doctors are paid

Private practitioners get paid a fixed sum for running their practice and also, like the GPs working at the health centres, monthly salaries according to a negotiated general contract. Additionally all GPs get a fee for service which is a relatively large part of their total salaries. No extra fee is paid for telephone consultations.

What patients pay

The patients now pay nothing to visit their GP and IKR 900 (about £9) when seeing other specialists. The patients also have to pay £3 for laboratory or X-ray investigations. The inhabitants are covered by the National Health Insurance which pays the rest of the real cost per visit or investigations, and all hospitalization.

Access to general practice

The patients are instructed to seek their own GP which guarantees good continuity of care. The consultation time is 15-20 minutes. The patients make an appointment by telephoning the receptionist at the health centre when they want to see their doctor. About 80% get their non-acute appointment time the same day and almost everyone within three days. Urgent consultations take place the same day.

Every GP has a telephone time from 30-60 minutes every day when the patients can call their doctor directly for renewal of prescriptions or some other health problems. The patients do not have to talk first to the nurse as in many other countries before they reach their GP by phone. The mean number of office consultations per GP is 240 consultations per month. Minor accidents are usually treated at the health centre.

Prevention and screening

Surveys in Iceland have shown that up to 90% of all inhabitants contact their health centre every year. The number of contacts averages about 6 per person per year. 35% of these contacts are by telephone. The high proportion of contacts and continuity of care gives the health personnel an exceptionally good opportunity for opportunist health promotion, case finding, advice about health seeking behaviour and other forms of instruction. As a result, the need for screening surveys may be reduced.

In most health centres GPs take care of maternity and child health care and the school health service. In some places they also look after the environmental and occupational health services. In Reykjavik and surroundings the maternal and child health care is organized in cooperation with specialists in obstetrics and paediatrics who see the mothers and children in accordance with a schedule. The obstetricians, for example, see every pregnant woman at the beginning and near the end of pregnancy; whereas the GPs, nurses and midwives take care of the other routine examinations as well as any other problems that might occur. GPs are not usually involved in deliveries and treatment in hospital, as in some other countries. The Icelandic College recommends that prevention, screening and medical care should be merged. For this purpose problem oriented medical records are necessary.

The potential of the consultation is stressed, and the use of health maintenance flow charts for case finding and screening is recommended. In this way, many of the preventive measures are built into the infrastructure of the health centre.

Computerization

An experiment was started in 1976 to evaluate problem oriented medical records (POMR) in primary health care and to computerize all the encounters in a systematic way. Some years later the Directorate of Public Health decided to use POMR all over the country and the use of personal computers has increased extensively. About 50% of health centres are using computers, although to a varying extent, and a program is being developed to computerize the whole medical record. 85% of the capital cost of computer equipment and programs has been financed by the state, the remainder and the running expenses being paid by the local authorities. However, after 1989 all the running expenses will be paid by the state.

Facilities available at health centres

All the health centres are equipped in accordance with standards recommended by the health authorities and the Icelandic College of Family Physicians. This includes, for example, ECG instruments, X-rays in some places, oto-microscopes etc, according to the type of service the centre aims to provide.

Alternative medicine

The Icelanders have strong beliefs in supernatural phenomena. The use of alternative therapies such as acupuncture, chiropractic, yoga and meditation is, however, not very common. According to a recent survey, 76% of those asked had used the health service for themselves or a relative during the previous three months, but only 10% had used alternative medicine during this time.

Referrals

Referral to a specialist by a general practitioner has not been mandatory in recent years, but the matter is being discussed by doctors and health authorities.

Special characteristics

The population of Iceland has a very high proportion of children and teenagers (30% of population are aged less than 16). 13% are over 60 (compared to 20% in Sweden). This means that Icelandic GPs deal with a lot of common children's diseases but relatively few geriatric problems. Icelanders are regarded as workaholics, so musculo-skeletal complaints are common.

In a Gallup poll of 27 countries in 1984, Icelanders seemed to be the most content with their state of life, and seemed to be the happiest people in the world. This may be true, but one of many possible explanations may be that they are not used to complaining, nor making a fuss about small things. To complain of tiredness, for example, seems ridiculous except after working for 24 hours.

Further reading

1. Annus Medicus public health report (1988) Health care in Iceland: the present situation and future goals. Directorate general of Public Health Reykjavik 1989.
2. Sigurdsson J et al (1988) Access to primary health care in urban Iceland. Scand J Prim Health Care 6:87-91.

Arrangements for vocational training of GPs

Dr Jóhann A Sigurdsson

Proportion of vocationally trained GPs

Since 1970, family medicine has been accepted as a specialty in Iceland. Out of a total of 150 GPs working in Iceland, there are now 67 doctors (45%) who have completed this vocational training. Almost every medical graduate goes abroad for further postgraduate education, mainly to USA and Sweden. Most of those who want to be GPs go to Sweden and Canada. About 35 doctors complete postgraduate education (in all kinds of specialties) every year. Of these there are about five doctors (15%) who specialize in general practice.

Length of vocational training

The trainee has to fulfil certain educational programmes which, since 1986, are as follows:

- Undergraduate medical education for six years.
- Clinical training spent at hospital for one year.
- Specialty in family medicine:

  a) Two years in general practice, placed at health centre with supervision of GP specialized in family medicine. Six months of this time can be changed to time spent in other disciplines such as otolaryngology, dermatology, anesthesiology, surgery and rehabilitation (or as in section C below), but not more than three months in each department.

  b) One year spent in internal medicine.

  c) 18 months total spent within pediatrics, psychiatry, gynaecology and obstetrics or surgery, with a minimal time of four months within each department.

  d) Instead of education according to a), b) and c) an organized vocational training in general practice/family medicine in other countries can be accepted. The time spent in vocation training however must be at least four years.

No final examination is required. As mentioned above, most of the Icelandic doctors get their postgraduate degree abroad.

The content of vocational training (tutorial methods)

This training programme is very similar to those in the other Nordic countries, because of an agreement between these countries of a common labour-market. As seen from above, the legislation only lays down the time spent in various departments and health centres and says nothing about the content of the training programme. However, the tasks for the GP and the objectives at the health centre are defined in the legislation on health care and furthermore The College of Family Physicians has published a report on standards in general practice. In this report certain factors are stressed such as a) education of the GP, b) facilities at his/her working place, and c) how he/she works.

These objectives can be used for the trainee, but further description, organisation and manpower is still missing for an effective vocational training in family medicine in Iceland.

Trainers and future plans

The Icelandic Medical Association is mainly responsible for the vocational training programmes together with the Faculty of Medicine, University of Iceland. There are at this moment two assistant professors (lecturers in British parlance) in family medicine who take care of the undergraduate education in family medicine. There are plans for a professorial chair in the discipline in the near future and he will then be involved in postgraduate training programmes.

Arrangements for continuing medical education of GPs

Dr Jóhann A Sigurdsson

Responsibility

The State, the College of Family Physicians and pharmaceutical firms are mainly responsible for CME.

Travel abroad

The Icelanders have since the country was settled in the eighth century been afraid of too much isolation. The original meaning of the word "heimskur" which means stupid, is 'the one who stays at home'. This is one of many explanations why the Icelanders stress the importance of experience and education abroad.

According to an agreement with the State, every doctor is allowed to travel abroad once in a year for 15 days for CME. The doctor can decide to which place he/she wants to travel, if it is within a reasonable distance. San Fransisco to the west and Tel Aviv to the south east have been used as reference distances. The doctor keeps his salary during this time and the State pays the travel expenses, possible congress or workshop costs and a certain amount for food and accommodation.

Meetings

The College arranges regular CME meetings once a month for GPs working in Reykjavik and the surrounding area. The meetings in other parts of Iceland are more sporadic. The GPs themselves are usually responsible for, and provide the main contribution to the programme. Furthermore there are about two or three symposia or workshops each year about topics which are highlighted such as hyperlipidaemias, computers in primary health care, etc.

Conferences

Conferences in general practice, held every second year by the Colleges of General Practice/Family Medicine in the Nordic countries, now play an important role for CME. The Icelandic Medical Association arranges annual postgraduate conferences for two or three days which usually are of some interest to the GPs.

Pharmaceutical input

Pharmaceutical firms play a part in CME in Iceland as in other countries. This is usually in the form of arrangement of evening sessions, visits by representatives to health centres once a week or by inviting individual doctors to conferences abroad. Some of the firms have offered services such as literature search etc. The Icelandic College of Family Physicians has published guidelines for GPs regarding professional cooperation with the pharmaceutical industry. It is difficult to say how large a part pharmaceutical firms play in CME and it varies greatly between individual doctors, probably in the range of 5-20% of all organized CME.

Further reading

1. Iceland 1986. Handbook published by the Central Bank of Iceland. Nordal J and Kristinsson V. (Eds). Reykjavik 1987.
2. Health Care in Iceland (1988). The present situation and future goals. Annus medicus public health report 1988. Director General of Public Health, Reykjavik. August 1989.
3. Palsdottir D (1989). Reviews. Ministry of Health and Social Security. Reyjkavik.
4. Sigurdsson JA, Johnsen S, Magnusson G. (1988). Access to primary health care in urban Iceland. Scand J Prim Health Care vol 6; 87-91.

Section 4
Norway : Norge

Demography and organization of health system

Dr Wenche Telstad

Demography

Population: 4.2 millions. Size: 386 958 km^2. Density 10.8/km^2. 16% of the population are over 65. 7% are over 75. Predictions of growth of the elderly population are lower than in other Nordic countries, with the exception of Iceland.

Norway extends from the level of Caithness in Scotland in the south, to the 71st parallel of latitude over 400km north of the Arctic Circle. It has boundaries with Sweden, Finland and Russia. The inhabited part of the island of Svalbard extends to the 80th parallel.

Health expenditure

The percentage of gross national product spent on health is 7% (1987). The percentage of the health budget spent on general practice is 5.6% (1987), and on primary health care 19.6% (1987).

Organization of health care

Up to 1984 Norway had a system of district physicians. These were doctors working part-time in community health, employed by the county, and part-time as self-employed private GPs. Since 1984 the municipality has taken over the responsibility for primary health care.

In every municipality there is a doctor responsible for medical services and community health. There are 448 municipalities. In the smaller places there is one chief of health and social service, and this is very seldom a doctor: more often a social worker or, for example, a teacher. In the bigger places there are two or three divisions: one for health, sometimes under the leadership of a doctor; one for social services; and one for nursing homes and home nursing, often headed by a nurse.

The hospitals are still under the counties, and there are a few State hospitals as well with more specialized services.

There were 3100 general practitioners in 1988: 2900 in 1987.

Health centres

The exact numbers of health centres is not known. They are very seldom administered as centres, but it happens that different kinds of service share the same building. There is seldom a close connection, but they cooperate as separate units. There is no common model for such centres. For example, my last place of work was a centre with three GPs, there was an office for home nursing; for a psychologist working in the schools; for the social security service; a centre for the elderly with a cafeteria; a pharmacist; a physiotherapist; and a library.

GPs commonly work together in such centres: specialists are rarely integrated in them. They are referred to as group practices. 30% of GPs work single-handed; 20% work in a group of two; 22% in a group of three; 11.5% in a group of four and the rest in bigger groups.

Staff

Most GPs employ secretaries. They have a one year training for work as medical secretaries. They are also trained in minor surgical and laboratory procedures, take ECG, blood tests etc. Some practices also have nurses or laboratory staff.

Consultations

The average length of a consultation is 15 minutes. Urgent cases are always seen the same day. Non-urgent cases may be seen the same day in outlying districts, but there may be a wait of up to 4-8 weeks in some of the bigger cities. The standards of the health service and availability of primary health care vary greatly depending on the resources available in the municipality.

Financial arrangements

There are different systems for employment and payment for GPs. One third are self employed and have an agreement with the municipalities. They get 30% from the social security, 40% from the municipality as a monthly payment and 30% from the patient. There are around 300 of the 'combined' physicians left - they have also a salary from the municipality for community health care. When a new GP appointment is made, this part of the job (and the salary) are lost. As a consequence, this group of doctors is getting smaller every year.

There are a few doctors, mostly in the bigger or central areas, with no agreement with the municipalities (or the counties for the specialists). They get their fees from the social security and from patients.

The social security system pays, at varying rates, for taking laboratory specimens as well as for tests done in the practice. Procedures such as audiometry, rectoscopy, tonometry and surgical procedures are paid for.

What patients pay

Patients pay Nkr 63 (£6) for each consultation with a GP, even a GP-specialist. Nkr 80 (£7) is paid to see a specialist. There is no charge for staying in hospital, but outpatients are charged. An operation may cost up to Nkr 880 (£80): an X-ray Nkr 80. Transport and medicines are paid for. Only a small percentage of the price of medicines for certain diseases is charged. These are written on a special card, and the patient pays up to Nkr 950 (£85), the remaining cost being paid by social security (one parent and all the children in a family may be grouped together). Patients pay for physiotherapy, except in certain diseases, when it is free.

Computerization

Of the GPs employed by municipalities, 17.4% have data systems. 25% of GPs in private practice with an agreement have a computer: 37.5% of those without an agreement. These practices have all been set up since 1984.

Use of laboratory, X-rays and ECG

Almost all GPs and practices have facilities for electrocardiography, simple blood tests such as haemoglobin and ESR, urine tests and microscopy. About 20% have equipment for serum analysis and cell counts. In outlying districts, practices commonly have X-ray facilities and a defibrillator.

Alternative therapy

Chiropractors are now approved by health authorities. There are some homeopaths with a three year training, but they are not officially approved. Acupuncture is not common, but some doctors and physiotherapists are qualified to do it. There are also zone-therapists, aromatherapists etc. The public use these services where they are available. In the bigger cities, up to 30% of the population have tried alternative therapies.

Prevention and screening

There is a common programme for vaccination and screening of all children up to 16 years, run by specially trained nurses and GPs. There is no official programme for screening adults. Cervical screening and mammography services are being planned but are not yet in operation. Some GPs have their own screening programmes, including people over 70. Some employers arrange for their employees to have an annual medical check.

Complaints procedures

All GPs should have a poster in their surgery telling the patient what to do when they wish to complain. The complaint should be sent to the head doctor in the municipality, or directly to the medical staff at county level. If the complaint is serious it is sent on to the Health Directorate and/or the Court. The patient may also contact a lawyer to have the case tried.

Data access and protection

Very strict laws regulate data protection in order to ensure secrecy of medical data. The patient (or patient's lawyer) has the right to see their own medical record. GPs do not have to supply copies, but this is usually done. Most commonly, the patient and GP read the records together so that technicalities can be explained. If patients think the records are inaccurate they may ask for them to be corrected, or complain about them.

Arrangements for secondary care

These are agreed between GPs and specialists. Referral is the norm, but it does not always happen, for example in an emergency. Some specialists do not bother about the agreement. Self-referral is uncommon, except with ophthalmologists, and perhaps in the case of home nursing where access to the general practitioner may not be so easy.

Medical manpower

The 'market' for doctors is regulated by laws passed in the last two years. New appointments, both in hospital and outside, must be approved by a regulatory board which aims to produce a stable medical structure, both of specialists and GPs. There is a shortage of trained nurses and physiotherapists in outlying hospitals. There is a national shortage of anaesthetists, neurologists, psychiatrists and radiologists.

Arrangements for vocational training of general practitioners

Professor John Maeland

Introduction

General practice was not established as a fully recognized specialty until 1985. Management of the vocational training programme is delegated to the Norwegian Medical Association. Of Norway's 2800 GPs, about 1800 are expected to have fulfilled the requirements for the specialty by 1990.

Length of vocational training

- General practice training: the trainees must spend 50% of their working hours in 'open, unselected clinical practice' during a four-year period.
- Hospital training: one year in a clinical department.
- Courses: at least 400 hours.
- Group-based general practice training programme: a two-year group-based educational programme consisting of 40 bi- weekly meetings.

Training/tutorial methods

Of the 400 hours of courses, 300 hours must cover mandatory issues. Four compulsory basic courses, each of 30 hours, cover the following topics: (1) general practice; (2) preventive medicine; (3) epidemiology and community medicine; and (4) practice management, health economics and law in medicine. The rest of the obligatory courses may be chosen from a large 'menu' of clinical topics.

Small-group learning

The group-based training programme is arranged as continuous study groups of 2 to 10 GPs headed by an appointed trainer. The groups meet regularly every two weeks for three-hour sessions. The topics cover clinical aspects, practical skills and the theoretical foundations of general practice. An Educational Handbook for General Practitioners presents introductory texts for the 20 recommended tutorials, with a selection of references for preparatory reading.

Training

The group members share the responsibility for the programme by conducting literature search, reading and introductory talks. Aspects of everyday practice work are recorded prior to some of the meetings, giving material for discussion. The aim is to create a continuous learning process in the groups, based on studying and professional feedback.

Teacher selection and training

The trainers are selected from experienced GPs, and a special programme for educating trainers has been developed, consisting of three one-week courses. The plan is to recruit 30 new trainers each year.

Assessment

There are no obligatory examinations. However, some of the theoretical courses include a brief pass or fail examination.

Arrangements for continuing medical education of GPs

Dr Jörund Straand

Re-certification of GP-specialists

Until recently, continuing medical education (CME) in general practice in Norway has been a loosely structured and voluntary activity. When general practice was established as a fully recognized specialty in 1985, rules for re-certification were also put into effect. Once recognized as a GP-specialist, re-certification is required every five years. General practice is currently the only specialty in Norway requiring re-certification.

Re-certification programme

This consists of three parts:

- Practice: at least 1 year of general practice during the five-year period.
- Course-hours: 200 hours required. All courses, both for the vocational training programme and for re-certification have to be approved by the Specialty Committee for General Practice of the Norwegian Medical Association. Courses arranged by pharmaceutical companies are not approved.
- Options: (1) At least three months practice at a hospital, or (2) at least one month of 'structured' hospital service (a structured clinical education programme within a certain clinical branch of hospital medicine. The programme is designed by hospital colleagues in collaboration with selected GPs), or (3) research in general practice for at least three months at one of the Institutes of General Practice, or (4) 100 more course-hours attending courses that are approved for general practice.

Leave of absence and financial costs

GPs employed by the municipal authorities can usually leave their practice for two weeks a year in order to take part in CME. GPs working on a fixed salary basis can keep their income during this two-week period.

The complete course programme, including travel and lodging is financed by the Postgraduate Education Fund of the Norwegian Medical Association.

The specialty of general practice is not obligatory for GPs practicing in Norway. However this postgraduate education is considered intellectually and professionally stimulating. Having completed the programme, the GP's wages as well as professional status are improved.

The specialty today and tomorrow?

The five year old programme for vocational training and re-certification is now under review. It is widely accepted by GPs in Norway that this programme has been a success. We do believe that the programme has become a useful tool to improve the quality of general practice. The task now is, therefore, not to change the programme radically, but to try to make a good programme even better.

Crucial questions

During the review, answers will be sought to the following questions:

- What should be the role, if any, of the Institutes of General Practice?
- Should there be examinations or not?
- Should courses within the re-certification programme be compulsory?
- Should hospital service be a compulsory part of the re-certification programme?
- Should re-certification of the specialty be mandatory throughout the professional lifetime?

Two important lessons

Up to now, two important lessons have emerged from the programme which might be of particular interest to colleagues abroad.

- Our experience supports the view that if one wants to educate general practitioners to handle the problems of general practice, this should take place in the setting of general practice and not in hospitals.
- Training for general practice can be organized differently from the the traditional one-to-one trainer-trainee model. The group-based and decentralized models provide a well-functioning setting for teaching and learning. The groups seem to facilitate the kind of professional feedback often lacking in general practice.

Further reading

1. Fugelli P, Hunshaar S, Maeland JG, Westin S. (1989) Training for general practice: a look to Norway. Family Medicine 21: 88-91, 150-1.

Section 5
Sweden : Sverige

Demography and organization of health system

Dr Christina Nerbrand

Demography

Population 8.5 million. Population over 65 (1985) 1.45 million: over 75 620,000, increasing to 890,000 by the year 2025. Life expectancy at birth (1985) 76.8 years. Land area 411 258 km^2, density 21 persons per km^2.

Health costs

9.1% of gross national product spent on health care. This sum has decreased in real terms since 1982. 23% of the health budget is spent on primary health care (PHC).

Health care organization

The Health and Medical Services Act of 1983 states that the aim of the health services is to provide good health care on equal terms for the entire population. The patient's right to participate in decisions about his or her medical care is well defined. The responsibility for organizing and providing primary and secondary health care rests with the local county council. Tertiary care is organized by six regional authorities. Regional hospitals also function as teaching hospitals. All health care is financed by taxation (apart from contributions by patients) and administered by locally elected bodies.

Primary health care organization

PHC is defined as the basic level of health care for the whole population. There are 850 health centres in Sweden each looking after a known population residing in a geographical area. PHC also covers district nursing, home care, preventive services, screening for risk factors, school health care, nursing homes and some long stay hospital care.

General practitioners

There are about 2800 GPs (about one per 3000 population). There is a shortage of GPs in some health centres, and recruitment is difficult in some areas. General practice has been regarded by entrants to the profession as having a lower status than hospital medicine, but this is changing.

Health centres

Most of the health centres have been built in the last 20 years and are very well equipped. They have been located more in rural areas and the big cities may lack the capacity for PHC. Paediatricians, gynaecologists and psychiatrists may also work in health centres, but do not have a strictly defined popoulation. Health centres vary in size from two to more than 10 doctors. The goal is to have one GP per 1500 - 2000 population.

Health centres have laboratory facilities and physiotherapy units. Physiotherapists also make home visits.

Staff and teamwork

GPs work with other professions in a health centre, for example district nurses, nursing aides, secretaries (in all 2 - 3 per GP), also with physiotherapists, paediatric nurses and midwives. GPs cooperate closely with welfare and social security authorities in their local community.

Consultations

Patients visit a GP on average 1.2 times per year, and the same to district nurses. The GP's other activities account for a similar number of consultations. Out-of-hours care is organized by groups of doctors. Consultations are at a health centre. Very few house calls are made. The average length of consultation is 10 - 20 minutes. Nurses are available for telephone advice.

Quality assurance

A number of experiments have been carried out under the auspices of SPRI (The Swedish Planning and Rationalization Institute). These have covered protocol development for management of certain diseases (eg hypertension, asthma and diabetes), with audit of adherence to the protocol and outcome. SPRI have also undertaken studies in patient satisfaction about the way they are treated and their needs considered, the information they are given, the physical facilities and their personal integrity.

How GPs are paid

All GPs employed by the county council are salaried and these are centrally negotiated for a 40-hour week. Extra money is available for additional hours worked. Very few GPs in Sweden have a private practice.

What the patient pays

Patients pay 30 - 60 SEK (£3 - £6) for each visit to the GP (less for visiting the nurse). This includes any tests or referral to hospital. Hospital stay costs 55 SEK per day. Prescribed drugs cost a maximum of 65 SEK (£6.50) each. Certain categories are exempt (eg drugs for diabetes or asthma).

Computerization

Some health centres have very sophisticated computer systems, but most do not. Major projects for developing computer systems for PHC are under way.

Complaints

The Medical Disciplinary Board, a government board not associated with either the professions or the administrative system of the health care, handles patients' complaints. If a doctor is found guilty a warning could be given or the licence to practice withdrawn. The patient is indemnified against court costs. 'No fault compensation' is in operation.

Alternative therapies

Interest in alternative therapies is growing, but only chiropractors are officially recognized and cooperate with the medical system.

Plans for the future

A major strategic reassessment of health care provision started with legislation in 1985 initiating the 'Health care in the 1990s' project (HS90), which envisaged an expansion and improvement of PHC services. These services had been shown to relieve pressure on emergency services. The aim was for highly competent staff to provide continuity of care in PHC, with an expansion of home care services as well as collecting and analysing local data for planning of health services.

Further reading

1. SPRI (1987) Some facts about health care in Sweden. Bo Soderholm (Ed). Swedish Planning and Rationalization Institute, Stockholm.
2. The National Board of Health and Welfare (1985) The Swedish Health Services in the 1990s. S-106 30 Stockholm.

Organization of health services - Sweden

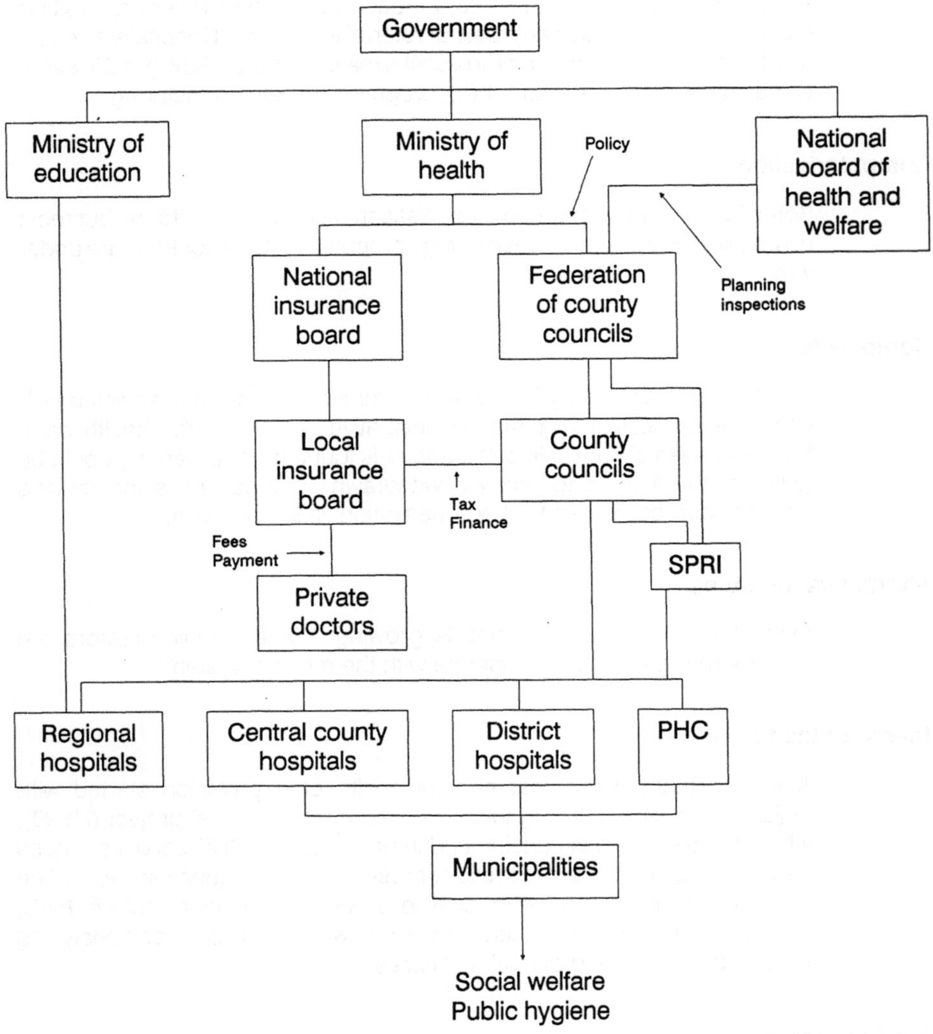

Arrangements for vocational training of general practitioners

Dr Bengt Mattsson and Dr Margareta Troein

Organization of vocational training

Of about 2800 general practitioners in Sweden, 2460 were members of the Association of General Practitioners (1989). 1902 were formally recognized as specialists in general practice. Each year, about 250 training posts are available. This number is less than it was three years ago, when there were about 350 training schemes.

Programmes

The training programme lasts four and a half years. Two of these years have to be spent in general practice, though six months can be interchanged with general surgery, orthopaedics, ear-nose-and-throat surgery or social/community medicine. Two and a half years are spent in hospital, one year in internal medicine, six months in psychiatry and four months in each of gynaecology, paediatrics and geriatrics.

A special training programme is worked out for each health centre. Around two thirds of the time is recommended to be spent in 'ordinary GP work' and one third of the time should be taken up with supervision, teaching, library studies and research. During the past years there has been a trend towards less work and more supervision. However, in practice, most GPs spend more time doing ordinary GP work. Many GP posts are vacant, particularly in the northern part of the country, so that trainees may sometimes find themselves doing full-time work.

Courses

Week-long courses are arranged by the National Board of Health, and these are called NLV-courses. Six have to be attended during the four and a half years of vocational training. This is compulsory. Every course ends with a short examination - written or oral. So six examinations must be passed in order to be recognized formally as a specialist in general practice. The six courses can be chosen from about eighty that are available. The trainee is recommended to take at least two courses focussed on general practice.

Trainers

An experienced GP is appointed as trainer for the whole period. Many trainees prefer to start with one year at the health centre, then the hospital phase, followed by another year at the same health centre.

Teaching methods

The training and tutorial methods vary a lot in different centres. Most trainees have a personal trainer at the health centre. One or two hours per week of personal supervision is usual. In most districts there are also lectures and group activities (Balint groups for example) and other kinds of education in which the trainee takes an active part.

Assessment

Apart from the tests at the end of each of the six NLV-courses, there is no formal examination. Once the four-and-a-half-years training has been completed according to the rules, recognition as a specialist in general practice follows. There is no re-certification in Sweden.

Teacher training

Teaching courses for trainers, of one week duration, have been organized since 1981 jointly by the County Councils (who are responsible for the health care system in each county) and the National Board of Health. About one thousand GPs have taken these courses - roughly half of the specialist GPs. The GPs interested in teaching have selected themselves by attending these courses. There are no statutory procedures for selecting trainers.

New initiatives

The need for additional training for the GP trainers has become apparent in the last few years. In some regions (Stockholm and northern Sweden for example) a new type of day-release training course has been developed. These have focussed on the role of supervisor. Further details can be obtained on application to the author.

University input

The University Departments of General Practice do not have a formal input into vocational training. However, many academic GPs are at the same time teachers at the NLV-courses. Some departments have their own NLV-courses with a more academic emphasis. It is now possible for trainees to spend some of their time in academic departments (usually six months as a research worker).

The future

Dr Margareta Troein

New legislation

Vocational training of general practitioners in Sweden will change within the next few years. Parliament recently passed legislation stating that specialist training will become target-oriented. As a consequence, the present system, with the necessary amount of training defined only by the numbers of months of service, will be ruled out. Instead, the training will be regarded as complete when the personal tutor considers certain preset goals to be fulfilled. This will take approximately five to six years, provided the trainee works full-time.

Role of trainer

The role of the trainer will become increasingly important in the future. At present there are no formal criteria for becoming a trainer, but voluntary one-week courses are offered. Hopefully, the new system will lead to the development of formal education of trainers. This would probably increase the appreciation among colleagues and staff of the importance of vocational training.

How to achieve goals?

The specific means to reach the preset goal are not legally stated. We expect an elaboration of goal systems and advice on possible ways to reach these goals. This will be carried out by the GPs' organizations by developing curricula. The implementation of these on the local level requires GPs to take on the role of local director of education, a person who knows all about the training potential available in primary health care and in the hospital. He or she must also have the formal authority to influence conditions of training.

Assessment

The trainer's position will be powerful as he or she is authorized to decide when training is complete. It is necessary for the trainee to be able to get an independent assessment in case the trainer's and the trainee's views of fulfilment of goals differ. The present development of a voluntary specialist examination with an independent board may provide trainees with the opportunity of this second opinion.

Arrangements for continuing medical education of GPs

Dr Bengt Mattsson

Attendance at 'external' CME

A survey among GPs in 1986 showed that each, on average, spent 3 - 4 full days per year on continuing medical education (CME) outside the health centres in the form of courses, seminars etc. In 1983 the average figure was higher - 5-6 days on external CME.

'Internal' CME

On the other hand, internal CME (within the health centre) has increased and currently receives more emphasis. A rough estimate shows that about one third of GPs very rarely, or never, attend officially recognized CME. About one third attend sometimes, and the remaining third are regular and frequent attenders.

Finance

Full salary, travel, course fees and residential expenses are paid for GPs attending CME sessions. However, the cost of a replacement is seldom met. Economic responsibility tends to be decentralized, and each health centre has its own budget. As a result, the kind of support given to CME may vary between different centres.

Teaching methods

Official sessions usually take the form of lectures or small group work. Lecturing is still the most common method, though alternative teaching methods are sometimes used.

Specialist input

For many years the so-called 'Fund of the GP's Association' has run 20 - 25 week-long courses for GPs every year. The courses are usually given by GP-orientated specialists who present up-to-date news from their specialty, for example obstetrics/gynaecology, dermatology, psychiatry and internal medicine. Courses on orthopaedic medicine are particularly popular among the 'Fund' courses.

Pharmaceutical firm input

The pharmaceutical companies have had an increased role in CME during the past years. Almost every month, one or two invitations arrive for GP courses, usually of one to two days and focussed on a clinical topic. Sometimes these are run jointly with the National GP Association.

Future trends

The GP Association's focus for the future is on increased local activity. They recommend regular meetings of one to two hours (or longer) at the local health centre. In addition, GPs are recommended to spend at least one half day a month on CME organized jointly by five to ten health centres in the local Health Region. There is also increasing interest in small group sessions of the 'Balint group' type, also held within the local region.

Section 6
United Kingdom

Demography and organization of health system

Professor James Knox and Dr Peter Pritchard

Demography

The UK population in 1988 was 57.07 million (Scotland 5.08m, N Ireland 1.57m). The population as a whole has expanded 1.4% between 1977 and 1988, but the population over 65 has expanded by 8.3%; the over 75s by 27,3%; and the over 85s by 41.6% during the same period. There are 3.9 million over 75s, amounting to 6.8% of the population. This demographic time bomb is on a short fuse, and poses a problem for health care, particularly primary health care (PHC) that has not been faced in UK (see figure 6.1.).

Life expectancy at birth (1987) is 72.1 years for males and 77.8 for females. (See tables of international comparisons at end). The land area is 244 000 km^2 (94 209 square miles) and the population density 234 per km^2.

Health expenditure

£24.8 billion was spent on the National Health Service (NHS) in 1989 (5.9% of the GNP). Private health expenditure was £1.8 billion, and other health expenditure (such as privately bought medicines) £2.2 billion. The total expenditure in 1989 (including contributions by patients) was £29.5 billion (6.89% of GNP), or £446 per head. Those over 75 account for 26% of NHS expenditure. In 1973 the figure was 21%. Adjustment for inflation shows that NHS expenditure has increased by about one quarter in real terms, whereas expenditure on private health care has doubled between 1973 and 1988.

The general practitioner service accounts for about 8% of NHS expenditure, all of which comes from central funds. Prescriptions cost a total of £2.527 billion, or about £44 per head, or £74 560 per GP (1988).

NHS organization

The Secretary of State for Health and the Department of Health are responsible for the NHS. Management decisions are channelled through the NHS Management Board to 14 Regional and 193 District Health Authorities (in England), each headed by a chairman or woman and a general manager. The arrangements in Wales, Scotland and Northern Ireland are slightly different. Health Authorities are mostly concerned with

Figure 7.1.

Population and vital statistics

UK population and projections, index 1948 = 100

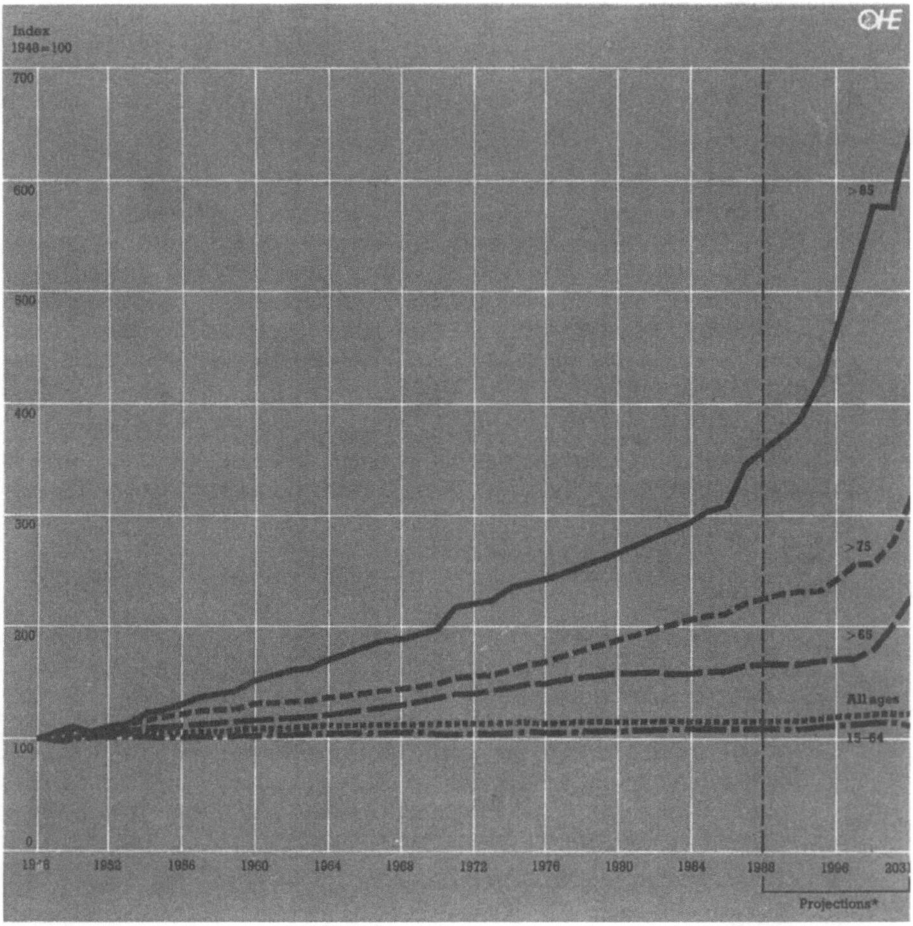

Note: *Projections based on 1987 mid-year estimates.

Source: Annual Abstract of Statistics.

From Compendium of Health Statistics, 7th Edition, 1989. Published by the Office of Health Economics, London. Reproduced by kind permission of the Director.

hospital services, though they do run the community nursing services and own health centres. On 1 April 1990 Regional Health Authorities will take overall responsibility for the GP services. They are already responsible for teaching.

Organization of general practice

GPs are independently in contract with the Secretary of State, via the Family Practitioner Committees (FPCs) in England and Wales (98 in all), and Health Boards in Scotland and Northern Ireland (19 in all). On 1 April 1990 a new contract will be imposed on GPs. FPCs will be restructured to give them greater powers of control over GPs and they will administer the contract and impose cash limits on GP spending. The new contract is a major departure from the previous 'laissez faire' approach, and is not popular with GPs. There are several features that will be very difficult to implement, and a large investment (more than £24 million) in information technology will be needed before it can function as planned. One good feature of the new contract is that some sort of quality assurance will be mandatory for all doctors. This has been a major objective of the Royal College of General Practitioners.

General practitioners

There were 34 495 GPs in UK in 1989, of whom 31 723 were 'unrestricted NHS principals' and 2279 were trainees. The total number of GPs had increased by 20% in the previous 10 years: the trainees had more than doubled in numbers. The distribution over the UK is fairly even, averaging about one unrestricted principal per 1800 population. (Some GPs are part-time or have limited lists.) The average list size of registered patients was 1913 in 1989 and lists are getting smaller. In Scotland the average list is 1584. GPs mostly work in partnership: only about one GP in 10 is single-handed and their numbers are diminishing. At present partnerships of 3 or 4 are the most popular, but the area of most rapid growth is in partnerships of 6 or more GPs.

Consultations

Patients consult their NHS GP about 4 times a year on average. In most practices, patients can get an appointment the same or the next day if they request it, but some GPs allow delays of up to a week to build up. This delay is not acceptable to most patients. The length of the consultation averages 8.25 minutes. Some GPs still book patients at 5 minute intervals, but the effectiveness of the consultation suffers. Many GPs try to include opportunistic screening when patients attend for other reasons. Other practices prefer to send for people by letter or to hold special well-person clinics. They are becoming popular, as are special sessions for diabetic and asthmatic patients.

Communication

All doctors entering practice have been trained in communication skills and are being encouraged to have explanatory leaflets for patients about the practice and how to obtain care. Some practices have newsletters with a strong emphasis on health promotion. A few practices (about 1.5%) have a 'patient participation group' in which GPs, staff and patients try to work as partners in improving the practice and improving patients' health. These activities are supported in the new contract.

Practice management

The development of larger practices with more variety of staff, and the complexity of the new contract, have made effective management essential. More practice managers are being recruited to take the administrative load off the GPs and to develop computerization. Practices will have to produce an annual report of their activities for the FPC, and this task will fall to the practice manager.

Computerization

GPs have always had to buy their own computer systems and software, and this has inhibited progress. In some areas one practice in three has a computer, in others the figure is two out of three and rising fast. The Government will contribute to costs, because a computer is essential to process the data required by the new contract. There is now strict data protection legislation in UK and all computerized practices need to be registered under the Act.

Clinical audit and quality of care

One of the main objectives of the new contract is to raise the standards of all practices to that of the best. Clinical audit will be obligatory, but how it will be achieved is unclear as yet. Many practices are doing this already, and one particularly successful method has been the 'Rent-an-Audit' system developed in Oxfordshire, which is now used by over 65% of practices in the county. The methods of practice assessment for the selection of teachers have also spread to non-teaching practices, but not so widely.

Prescription audit is being strengthened. GPs now receive details of their prescribing behaviour and costs every 3 months. From 1 April 1991 it will be monthly.

Diagnostic and other services

Laboratory services are very rarely located in primary health care, so patients usually have blood specimens taken by the GP or practice nurse and sent to the laboratory, often by NHS transport. For X- rays, the patient must usually be referred to hospital, particularly for contrast studies. Open access by GPs to endoscopy services is spreading and has been shown to be cost effective.

Very few practices have physiotherapy or occupational therapy on the premises. Psychologists and counsellors are increasingly working in primary health care, but their numbers are few.

Premises

Most GPs now work from purpose-built premises which they own, with 30% based on State-owned health centres. Many of the premises have space for attached district nurses and health visitors. The 'notional rent' of the premises is fully reimbursed by the FPC.

Staff and teamwork

All GPs now have the rudiments of a team, including secretary/receptionists and nurses. Many GPs now employ practice nurses, particularly to handle the increase in preventive work in the new contract. 70% of staff salaries are reimbursed by the FPC up to a limit of two full-time staff per GP, but this is threatened under the new contract.

Most GPs work in conjunction with district nurses and health visitors employed by the health authority. These nurses have a high degree of professional autonomy and owe their allegiance primarily to the patient. Some practices have well-developed teams with social workers and other health professionals, but the general level of teamwork lags far behind the best.

Payment of the GP

Nearly half the GP's NHS income comes from 'allowances' which are like a salary. The remainder is dependent on the number of patients on the list (capitation), plus fees for certain items of service such as immunization, cervical cytology and seeing temporary residents etc. The new contract aims to increase the capitation element from the present average of 46% of NHS income to at least 60%. This will give GPs a financial incentive to have larger lists of patients.

GPs' average NHS income is currently around £45 761, but £14 656 is intended for expenses, leaving an intended net pay of £31 105 per annum before tax (top rate 40%). Practice income varies widely, with many GPs earning more than £40 000. It would appear that GPs who spent as little as possible on staff and equipment would be better off. But studies have shown that GPs in well equipped and staffed premises and offering a wide range of services do, in fact, earn more. The new contract aims to reward those who reach prevention targets with an additional £5000 per annum - at the expense of the GPs who do not.

GPs can charge for work that comes outside their NHS duties, such as extra certificates and insurance examinations. The income from these services is small (less than 5%). One quarter of GPs are paid for doing hospital, school or factory sessions. They may take on private patients who are not on the their own list nor their partners'. For most practices it is a very small source of income.

What patients pay

There is no charge for seeing a GP, nor for hospital outpatient or inpatient care (with the small exception that some State benefits may be reduced while in hospital). Prescriptions are given free, but the patient has to pay £3.20 per item to the pharmacist. There are so many exemptions, that only 17% of items are paid for. Patients now have to pay for eye tests, and most of the cost of spectacles and dental treatment. Apart from these charges, the NHS is a free service, so that medical costs of illness are not a burden.

Complaints

People hold their GPs in high regard, and opinion polls and surveys have shown that around 90% of patients are satisfied with the care they receive, and around 80% of patients trust doctors - a far higher score than any other group. Politicians were only trusted by 5% of those polled. Complaints are few but are increasing. Mostly they are about the GPs manner and about refusing to visit the home when requested. Very few are about lack of technical competence.

Alternative therapies

These are very popular among those who can afford to pay for them. Virtually none are available under the NHS, with the exception of meditation, hypnosis, acupuncture and homoeopathy in a few centres. To some extent the demand for these therapies reflects people's perceived need for supernatural help (as confirmed by the national addiction to horoscopes). But they are also a measure of the inability of formal health care to give the amount of time and the kind of help that people feel that they need. GPs are becoming increasingly tolerant of alternative therapies and more willing to cooperate with the less bizarre varieties.

Private practice

As mentioned above, there is very little private general practice, but the hospital private sector is growing. This is partly a result of increasing waiting lists for non-urgent operations, and partly that more employees are being offered health insurance as a 'fringe benefit'. More than two million families (6 million people) in UK subscribe to these schemes - a sevenfold increase in 30 years.

'Internal market'

Under the new contract, the larger general practices may choose to have a budget for buying in secondary care (akin to the 'voucher' scheme pioneered in Scandinavia). This would include private care, which, if it were competitive on cost and quality, could obtain a larger share of the market. Doubts have been expressed about the viability of this concept of the 'internal market' in a situation in which there is no spare capacity; and also about the possibility of a 'two-tier' service developing. This has not happened so far in 40 years of the NHS which has been characterized by its popularity and its equity.

Some trends

The role of the GP as the traditional 'family doctor' is likely to continue, but the Government is placing more emphasis on 'pro- active' anticipatory care, health promotion, disease prevention and screening. GPs do not have a lot of spare time, so other activities may suffer, such as the care of the elderly and chronic sick, and activities outside the NHS.

The role of managers is being strengthened and this may curtail the GP's professional freedom. Consumer pressure is building up and this is sharpening the conflict between demand rather than need for health care on the one hand; and on the other hand the limited resources available. The British NHS is one of the cheapest in Europe, but is it adequate; is it good value for money; and will it be able to cope with the demographic time bomb?

The key question, in the light of experience from Nordic countries, is whether the level of investment of resources in PHC, as against secondary and tertiary care, is appropriately balanced.

Further reading

1. OHE Compendium of Health Statistics 7th edition 1989. Office of Health Economics, London SW1A 2DY

Arrangements for vocational training of GPs

Dr John Horder

Introduction

In 1989 there were 34 495 GPs in UK providing primary medical care within the NHS.[1] The number practicing outside the NHS is very small (probably less than 500).

Vocational training of 3 years duration became mandatory in 1980 for those wishing to practice as 'principals' in the NHS. This followed five and a half years of undergraduate medical education and one year of obligatory hospital appointments before registration as a doctor. But many entrants had completed this full programme voluntarily between 1970 and 1980.

Before 1970, some training was undertaken voluntarily by the majority of entrants, usually in hospital posts, but also in a training practice (the one-year 'trainee assistant' scheme started with the NHS in 1948). Only 10% of entrants to general practice between 1950 and 1970 totally lacked postgraduate hospital experience.

Numbers trained

The proportion of all GPs who have completed the 3 years of vocational training can only be estimated, but it is about 40%. In the last 5 years the average number of doctors accepted for the 3-year vocational training has been 2250 per year.

Training requirements

Of the three mandatory years, one must be spent in a selected training practice, and two in hospital or community medicine posts relevant to general practice. Most posts are of 6 months duration. Two must be chosen from among general medicine, paediatrics, geriatric medicine, psychiatry, obstetrics or gynaecology. A weekly day- or half-day-release course is available in every training scheme, sometimes continuing throughout the three years.

Training methods

Clinical responsibility under supervision occupies about 80% of the working time. In hospital posts this may be a higher proportion: in the training practices a smaller proportion, where there is regular individual tuition and also more opportunities to attend training courses which meet particular needs.

The training programme or syllabus varies from place to place, allowing for the initiative of course organizers and trainers. But the requirements for the examination for membership of the Royal College of General Practitioners (RCGP) exert their influence nationwide, ensuring a broad measure of conformity.

Whereas undergraduate medical education in UK has been moving to become an academic preparation for a changing future, the vocational training of GPs is centred on the job and uses the learner's practical experience as a basis. At its best, vocational training aims to meet and also to influence the individual learner's needs.

Assessment methods

The trainee has to secure a certificate of satisfactory completion at the end of each part of the 3-year sequence, from the person to whom she or he is immediately responsible. Refusal occurs, but infrequently.

At the end of vocational training, a trainee can take the examination for membership of the RCGP. Whereas the training is obligatory, the examination is not. The majority take it nevertheless, if only because there is now strong competition for permanent posts in general practice. The pass rate for trainees varies between 73% and 80%. The examination consists of multiple choice questions, an essay, 'modified essays' (progressive case-histories posing problems for resolution) and two viva-voce examinations. Bringing patients to the examination has not proved possible, but one of a pair of examiners often simulates a patient.[3]

Re-assessment

There is no re-assessment or re-certification of trainees. Trainers, however, have to be re-selected every 2 - 5 years (this varies from region to region). Fellowship of the RCGP (as distinct from membership), hitherto by recommendation, will in future be given only after a very exacting programme of performance review for those who offer themselves.

Trainers

There are more trainers approved than are needed each year. 3198 were approved in 1987. They are paid (currently £3870 per annum) only when they have responsibility for a trainee.

Selection of trainers

GP trainers are selected by methods that have become increasingly demanding. They are expected to have undertaken a teacher's course before applying. They are interviewed and their practice is always visited. In some regions the work of the practice may be observed in action and videotaped consultations inspected. Trainees are required to report on their training at the end of the year.[4,5]

Organization

Training in a region is controlled by a 'regional adviser' who holds a half-time university appointment. A national committee organizes visits of inspection. Regional advisers, course organizers, trainers and trainees all receive payment. Trainers meet regularly in local groups under a 'course organizer'.

University input

University departments of general practice - now in every medical school - exist primarily to teach undergraduate students, to initiate research and to contribute in various ways to the work of the medical school. Vocational training is organized and financed separately. The extent and form of the contribution made to vocational training by professors and lecturers varies from university to university.

At least four of the 26 medical schools have recently initiated master's (MSc) courses in general practice, lasting 2 years.

Future plans

The problems of protecting trainees in hospital posts from excessive clinical work, and of providing training appropriate to this stage - whether by the bedside, in tutorials, lectures or seminars - are not everywhere resolved. Obstetric posts give most difficulty. An increased element of education at this stage is nevertheless now national policy.

The standard of training practices is still too variable, despite steady improvement under a national system of inspection. In recent years it has been difficult for all who so choose to find places in vocational training schemes.

Styles[6] has recently suggested that vocational training must now pay increased attention to (i) a population-based approach, by teaching such skills as the collection and analysis of data; (ii) performance review; and (iii) practice management.

He also points out that the knowledge and skills required for general practice are difficult to contain within a three-year programme. Young principals both need and want to continue the sorts of learning to which they are now accustomed in vocational training, in their first years of unsupervised practice.

Summary

For all its problems, the vocational training scheme has been an outstanding success and the major influence in changing the face and the quality of general practice in UK. However, the process is a slow one, and only the start of a lifelong process of education which is considered in the next section.

References

1. Office of Health Economics (1989) Compendium of Health Statistics 7th edition. Office of Health Economics, London.
2. Department of Health and Social Security (1972). Enquiry into the previous medical experience of doctors joining the general medical services for the first time. Reports on Health & Social Subjects No 2. Her Majesty's Stationery Office, London.
3. RCGP. Explanatory notes for the MRCGP examination. Obtainable from the College, 14 Princes Gate, London SW7 1PU.
4. Joint Committee on Postgraduate Training for General Practice. (1985) Recommendations to regions for the establishment of criteria for the approval and re-approval of trainers in general practice. Obtainable from the Committee at 14 Princes Gate (see above).
5. Schofield TPC and Hasler JC. (1984) Approval of trainers in the Oxford Region: criteria. Brit. Med. J. 288 538-40, and 612-4.
6. Styles W. (1989) Tomorrow's general practitioners: preparing for change. In Managing to be a better doctor, MSD Foundation, Tavistock House South, London WC1H 9LG.

Arrangements for continuing medical education of GPs

Dr John Horder

Introduction

Continuing education in the United Kingdom is a voluntary activity, but one which is expected of every doctor. The provision is copious for those who seek it, especially in large cities. There have been several studies aiming to discover why some doctors make much more use than others of what is offered.[1,2,3,4,5]

Purpose

Keeping up to date is only one of the purposes of continuing education. Equally important are the stimulation of the GP's own thinking about common problems (both clinical and organizational); the maintenance of self-confidence and enthusiasm; and helping to overcome the still prevalent feeling of isolation. Specialists can help GPs to be aware of recent changes in their own specialty, but they can also act as a valuable resource in group discussions about general practice problems.

Provision and uptake

Most district general hospitals have created 'postgraduate centres' in the past thirty years, with lecture and seminar rooms, and provision for social contact. They are intended equally for the use of junior and senior hospital staff, as well as for GPs and sometimes other staff such as nurses. They have a particular value as places where GPs and specialists can meet.

In-house learning

In the last fifteen years, group practices have increasingly organized educational events on their own premises.[5,6] This has been encouraged by a trend, particularly among younger doctors, to prefer small-group work based on topical or practical problems, with the GPs themselves actively engaged both as learners and teachers.

Distance learning

Recently there has been extensive development of distance learning, using tapes, videos and television - especially popular among those who practice at a distance from teaching centres. This method is valuable also because it is available in the home or place of work, and is therefore time-saving.[7]

Organization of CME

Formal, official educational activities attract reimbursement of expenses under the National Health Service (NHS): what doctors organize for themselves has not, in the past. However, the distinction is an artificial one. Any statement about the official events neglects equally important methods like reading journals and individual case discussions with a specialist colleague. Nevertheless, it seems probable that those who attend more meetings are also those who make more use of other methods. Certainly, those who attend the popular lunch-time meetings, also attend more evening and weekend meetings.[3,4]

Uptake of CME

National figures were maintained by the Department of Health until 1976. Evidence from two studies, both from the north of England and not very recent are shown below:

Proportion of GPs who attended official half-day sessions per year:

	reference[1]	reference[2]
No sessions at all	4% of GPs	18% of GPs
1 - 15 sessions	78% of GPs	57% of GPs
more than 15 sessions	18% of GPs	25% of GPs

Financial arrangements

For many years the arrangements were generous, covering travel, subsistance and course expenses such as speakers, so that a GP could attend a course anywhere in the UK without cost. In the past ten years various limits have been imposed, although the basic system was unchanged.

Postgraduate education allowance (PGEA)

From now onward the system will be different. GPs will get a postgraduate education allowance (currently £1700 per annum) on condition that they produce evidence that they have attended five days of training per year, averaged over a five-year period. In those five years, at least two courses must be taken in health promotion and illness prevention, two in disease management, and two in service management. This represents an increase in control, but many details remain to be settled.

Training must be approved in order to qualify for the PGEA. The Committee of Regional Advisors in England has produced a list of ten criteria for approval. These include: the naming of an organizer for each activity who must state the aims of the activity and its relevance of the content to the learning needs of GPs and to services to patients; that the learning methods should be participative and active; that arrangements for evaluation and feedback should be specified; and that external assessment be allowed.

Role of pharmaceutical companies

Pharmaceutical companies frequently support CME, typically by providing food at a lunch-time meeting, but sometimes by much larger subsidies for a whole conference, when the importance of the event justifies this. Existing activities would be difficult to sustain without such help. Direct advertising of products tends to be more limited. Companies now set greater value on their name being associated with worthwhile events.

Future needs for CME

In the face of the vast range of possible topics, there is a need, firstly to move as far as possible towards agreement about those topics which are most essential and may even require frequent repetition (for example about common pitfalls in clinical practice, or about the management of emergencies); and secondly, in contrast, to identify those areas in which an individual doctor requires more knowledge and skill.

In reality, it is easier for both organizers and attenders to choose topics in which they are already interested (and therefore probably strongest). But if improved quality of care is the aim, then perhaps topics should be chosen which are not so interesting to attenders.[8] Self-assessment tests are, therefore, needed in order to find personal areas of weakness. 80% of GPs are willing to do them, but there is no information about how many actually carry them out. Performance review, self-initiated or with colleagues, can serve the same purpose.

Effectiveness of CME

Most people believe that CME is effective in improving the quality of care, but this is not easy to demonstrate. Few well- controlled studies have been done, and by no means all are positive. To take one review as an example, of 248 articles on studies of educational interventions, only 35 were about randomized controlled trials, and only three considered health outcomes for patients. There were significant benefits to patients in one of these three studies, but not in the other two. Several of these and other studies did, however, show improvement in the performance and competence of physicians.[9] The links between education, competence, performance and patient outcomes is therefore wide open for study.

Re-licensure

In the United States members of the Academy of Family Practice have grasped the nettle of re-licensure. In the UK the only approach has been in the new requirements for Fellowship of the Royal College.

References and further reading

1. Wood J and Byrne PS. (1980) Section 63 activities. Occasional paper No 11. Royal College of General Practitioners (RCGP), London.
2. Reedy BLEC. (1979) General practitioners and postgraduate education in the Northern Region. Occasional paper No 9. RCGP, London.
3. Pickup AJ, Mee LG, Hedley AJ. (1983) The general practitioner and continuing education. J. Roy. Coll. Gen. Practit. 33 486-490.
4. Branthwaite A et al. (1988) Continuing education of general practitioners. Occasional paper No 38. RCGP, London.
5. Owen PA et al. (1989) General practitioners' continuing education within and outside their practice. Brit. Med. J. 299 238-10.
6. Reiss BB et al. (1981) Practice educational meetings: a new influence in general practice. Brit Med. J. 283 1025-7.
7. Stott P, (1988) Distance learning, an increasingly important resource. Horizons 2(3) 129-131.
8. Sibley JC et al. (1982) A randomized trial of continuing medical education. New Eng. J. Mrd. 306 511-5.
9. Haynes RB et al. (1984) A critical appraisal of the efficacy of continuing medical education. J.A.M.A. 251 61-4.
10. Wood J (1988) Continuing education in general practice in the UK: a review. Family Practice. vol 5: 62-67. This up-to-date review is strongly recommended.

Section 7
Figures and Tables

Table 7.2

Population and vital statistics

OECD population (millions)

	1950	1960	1970	1975	1980	1985	1990e	1995e	2000e	2010e	2020e	2025e
Total OECD	**563.87**	**640.67**	**704.43**	**750.71**	**780.35**	**805.05**	**829.41**	**853.69**	**876.57**	**912.95**	**943.05**	**955.53**
Australia	8.22	10.32	12.55	13.63	14.70	15.70	16.71	17.69	18.63	20.32	21.89	22.58
Austria	6.94	7.05	7.45	7.52	7.51	7.50	7.51	7.52	7.52	7.45	7.36	7.28
Belgium	6.64	9.15	9.64	9.80	9.85	9.90	9.95	9.97	10.01	10.03	10.05	10.05
Canada	13.74	17.91	21.41	22.73	24.09	25.43	26.75	27.92	28.93	30.74	32.53	33.26
Denmark	4.27	4.58	4.93	5.06	5.12	5.12	5.12	5.11	5.08	4.97	4.80	4.69
Finland	4.01	4.43	4.61	4.71	4.78	4.89	4.97	5.02	5.06	5.07	5.04	4.99
France	41.74	45.68	50.67	52.71	53.71	54.62	55.48	56.34	57.16	57.93	58.35	58.43
W Germany	49.99	55.43	50.70	61.83	61.57	60.88	60.33	59.98	59.48	57.20	54.66	53.49
Greece	7.57	8.33	8.79	9.05	9.64	9.88	10.08	10.27	10.44	10.64	10.74	10.79
Iceland	0.14	0.18	0.20	0.22	0.23	0.24	0.25	0.27	0.27	0.29	0.30	0.30
Ireland	2.97	2.83	2.95	3.21	3.40	3.61	3.84	4.08	4.32	4.76	5.16	5.33
Italy	46.77	50.22	53.57	55.83	57.07	57.30	57.56	58.09	58.64	58.44	57.50	57.18
Japan	83.63	94.10	104.33	111.53	116.81	120.74	123.87	126.78	129.73	133.05	132.61	132.08
Luxembourg	0.30	0.31	0.34	0.36	0.36	0.36	0.36	0.36	0.36	0.35	0.34	0.34
Netherlands	10.11	11.48	13.03	13.79	14.15	14.50	14.75	14.96	15.08	15.06	14.86	14.69
New Zealand	1.91	2.37	2.82	3.09	3.17	3.32	3.46	3.61	3.75	3.97	4.14	4.20
Norway	3.27	3.58	3.88	4.01	4.09	4.14	4.18	4.20	4.22	4.23	4.26	4.26
Portugal	8.41	8.83	8.63	9.43	9.88	10.21	10.54	10.89	11.21	11.74	12.17	12.33
Spain	27.87	30.30	33.78	35.60	37.43	38.54	39.75	41.01	42.24	44.13	45.39	45.98
Sweden	7.01	7.48	8.04	8.19	8.31	8.35	8.31	8.24	8.17	8.00	7.82	7.71
Switzerland	4.70	5.36	6.27	6.41	6.33	6.37	6.39	6.38	6.34	6.16	5.92	5.78
Turkey	20.81	27.51	35.32	40.03	44.47	49.29	54.65	60.04	65.35	76.01	86.74	91.93
UK	50.62	52.56	55.48	56.04	55.95	56.13	56.19	56.31	56.35	56.13	56.08	55.92
USA	152.27	180.67	205.05	215.97	227.74	238.02	248.43	258.65	268.24	286.29	304.36	311.94
OECD elderly persons (over 65 years) expressed as % total population												
OECD average*	8.1	9.0	10.0	10.8	11.6	11.6	12.3	12.8	13.3	14.2	16.5	17.6
Australia	8.1	8.5	8.3	8.7	9.6	10.1	10.8	11.2	11.3	12.0	14.6	15.9
Austria	10.4	12.0	14.1	15.0	15.5	14.1	14.7	15.0	15.1	16.7	18.4	19.7
Belgium	11.1	12.0	13.4	13.9	14.3	13.4	14.3	15.1	15.8	15.8	18.3	19.8
Canada	7.7	7.5	7.9	8.5	9.7	10.4	11.3	11.9	12.2	13.4	16.9	18.8
Denmark	9.1	10.6	12.3	13.4	14.4	14.9	15.4	15.4	15.4	17.5	21.2	22.2
Finland	6.7	7.2	9.2	10.6	12.0	12.3	13.0	13.7	14.1	15.4	19.9	21.0
France	11.4	11.6	12.9	13.5	14.0	12.4	13.0	13.9	14.7	14.8	18.0	19.3
W Germany	9.4	10.8	13.2	14.3	15.5	14.5	15.1	15.8	16.7	20.0	21.2	22.5
Greece	6.8	8.3	11.1	12.2	13.1	13.1	13.4	14.7	16.1	16.7	17.2	17.8
Iceland	7.7	8.0	8.9	9.2	9.9	9.9	10.3	10.8	11.2	11.7	14.8	17.0
Ireland	10.7	11.2	11.2	11.0	10.7	10.4	10.1	9.5	9.1	8.9	10.6	11.0
Italy	8.3	9.3	10.7	12.1	13.5	13.0	14.1	15.1	16.1	17.2	18.8	19.6
Japan	4.9	5.7	7.1	7.9	9.0	10.0	11.4	13.2	15.1	18.0	20.8	20.3
Luxembourg	9.8	10.6	12.5	13.1	13.5	12.7	13.0	14.1	15.2	16.9	19.7	21.3
Netherlands	7.7	9.0	10.2	10.9	11.5	11.8	12.6	13.1	13.7	15.6	20.2	22.2
New Zealand	9.0	8.6	8.5	8.7	10.0	10.4	10.8	11.1	10.9	11.9	14.7	16.3
Norway	9.7	11.1	12.9	13.7	14.8	15.5	16.2	16.0	15.3	15.4	18.9	20.2
Portugal	7.0	8.0	9.7	9.9	10.5	10.5	11.1	11.8	12.3	12.4	14.3	15.7
Spain	7.3	8.2	9.8	10.0	10.7	11.1	11.7	12.6	13.6	13.8	14.7	15.7
Sweden	10.3	12.0	13.7	15.1	16.3	16.9	17.7	17.6	17.2	18.7	21.8	22.2
Switzerland	9.6	10.1	11.4	12.6	13.8	14.0	14.8	15.7	16.7	19.6	22.9	23.8
Turkey	3.3	3.5	4.4	4.5	4.6	4.2	4.2	4.9	5.5	6.1	7.3	8.4
UK	10.7	11.7	12.9	14.0	15.1	15.1	15.6	15.5	15.3	15.7	17.8	18.7
USA	8.1	9.2	9.8	10.5	11.3	11.7	12.2	12.3	12.0	12.3	15.4	17.2

Source: World Population Prospects, United Nations.

Notes: e = UN projections.
* Weighted average.

Figure 7.2.

Population and vital statistics

Sex differential in life expectancy (females less males) in OECD countries, 1985-1990

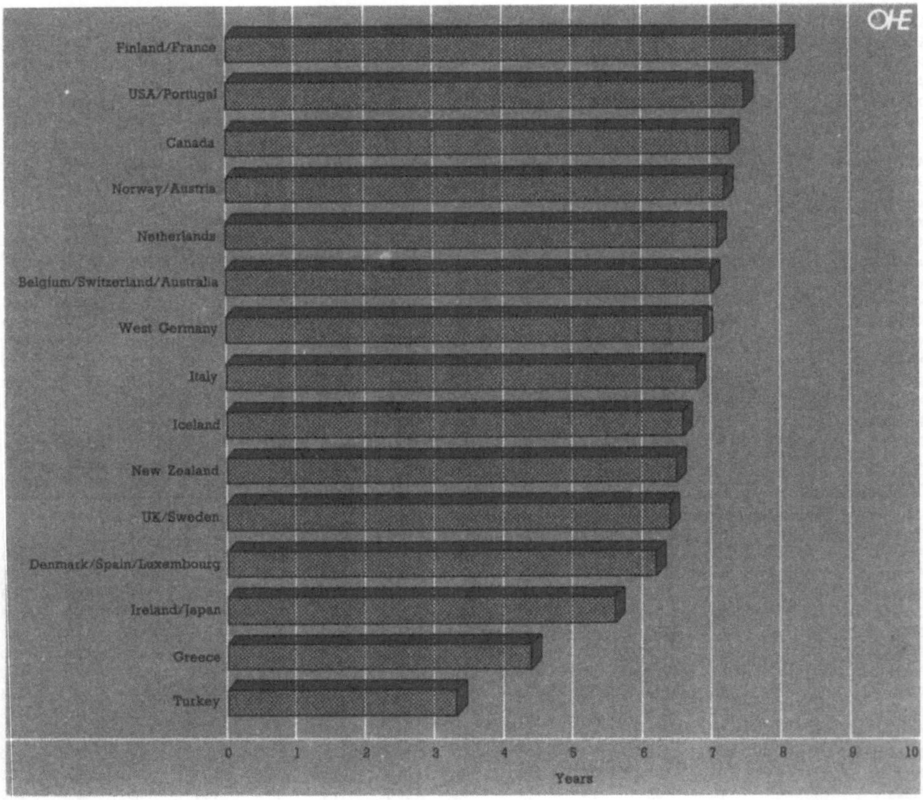

Source: United Nations.

From Compendium of Health Statistics, 7th Edition, 1989. Published by the Office of Health Economics, London. Reproduced by kind permission of the Director.

Figure 7.3.

Total health care expenditure

Relationship between health expenditure as per cent of GNP* and GNP* per head, 1987

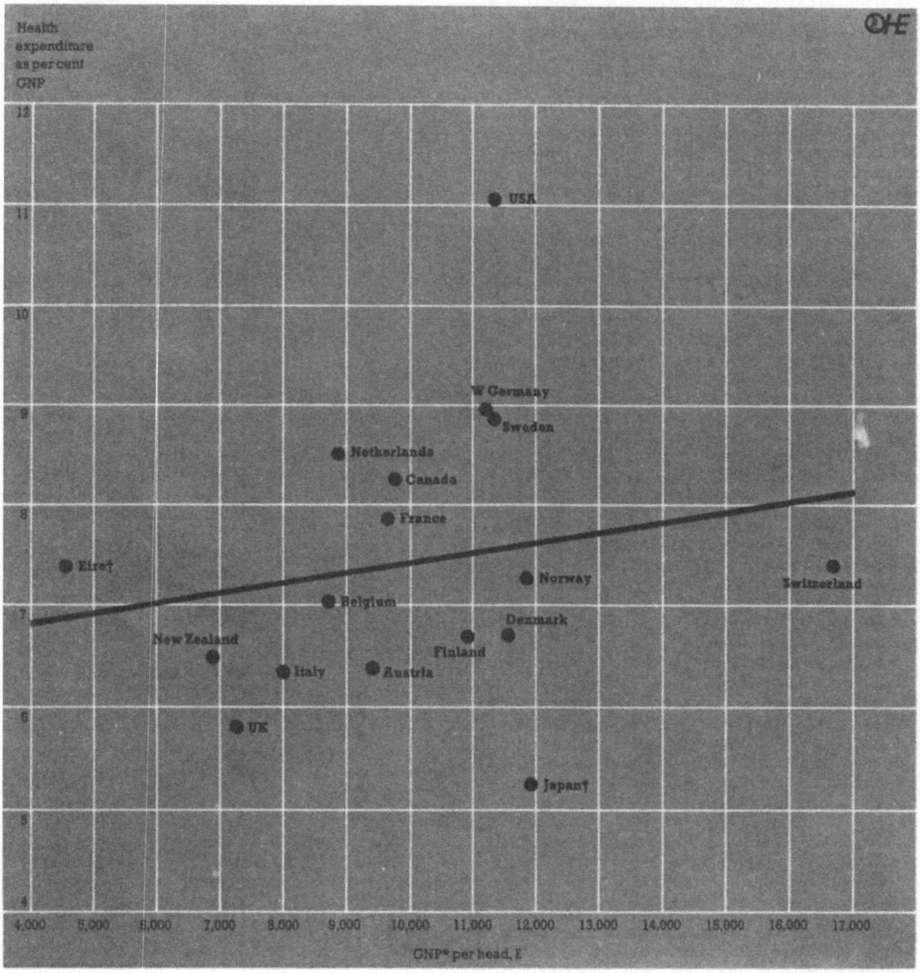

Notes: *Gross National Product at market price.
†Excluding private health expenditure.

Sources: OHE and IMF.

From Compendium of Health Statistics, 7th Edition, 1989. Published by the Office of Health Economics, London. Reproduced by kind permission of the Director.

Figure 7.4.

Total health care expenditure

Health expenditure* per person in selected OECD countries, 1987

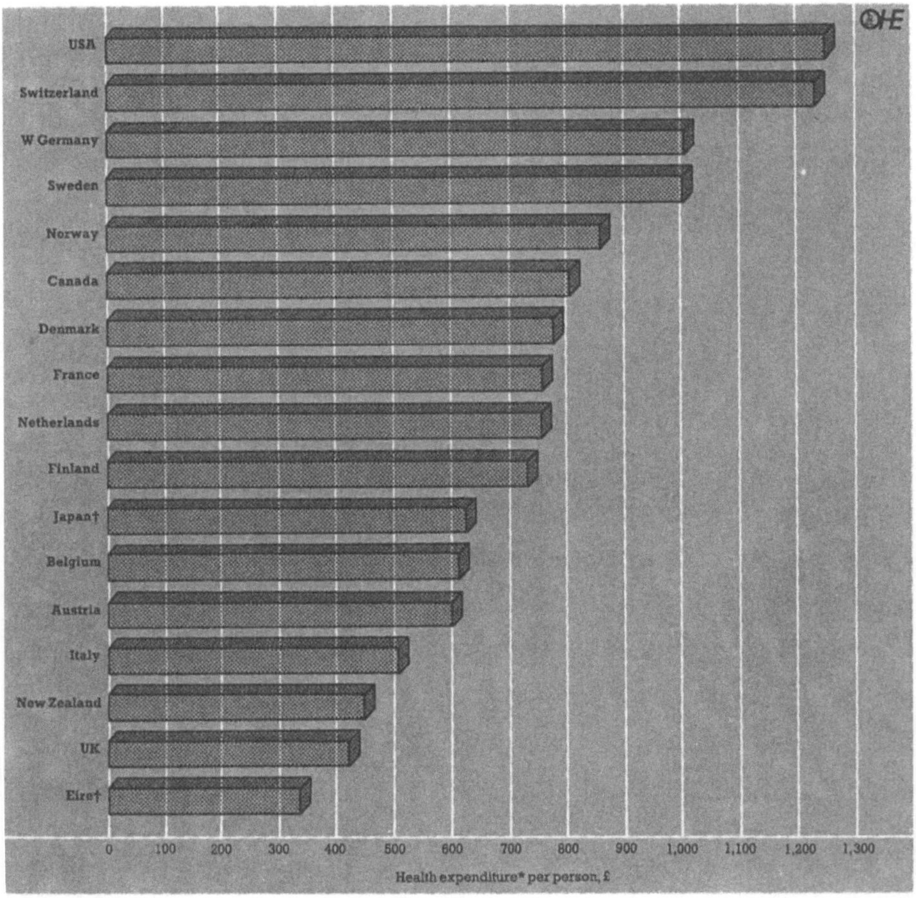

Notes: *Figures relate to public and private health expenditure.
†Figures relate to public expenditure only.

Source: OHE - private communications.

From Compendium of Health Statistics, 7th Edition, 1989. Published by the Office of Health Economics, London. Reproduced by kind permission of the Director.

Figure 7.5.

Pharmaceutical services

Per capita pharmaceutical consumption at manufacturers' prices, 1987

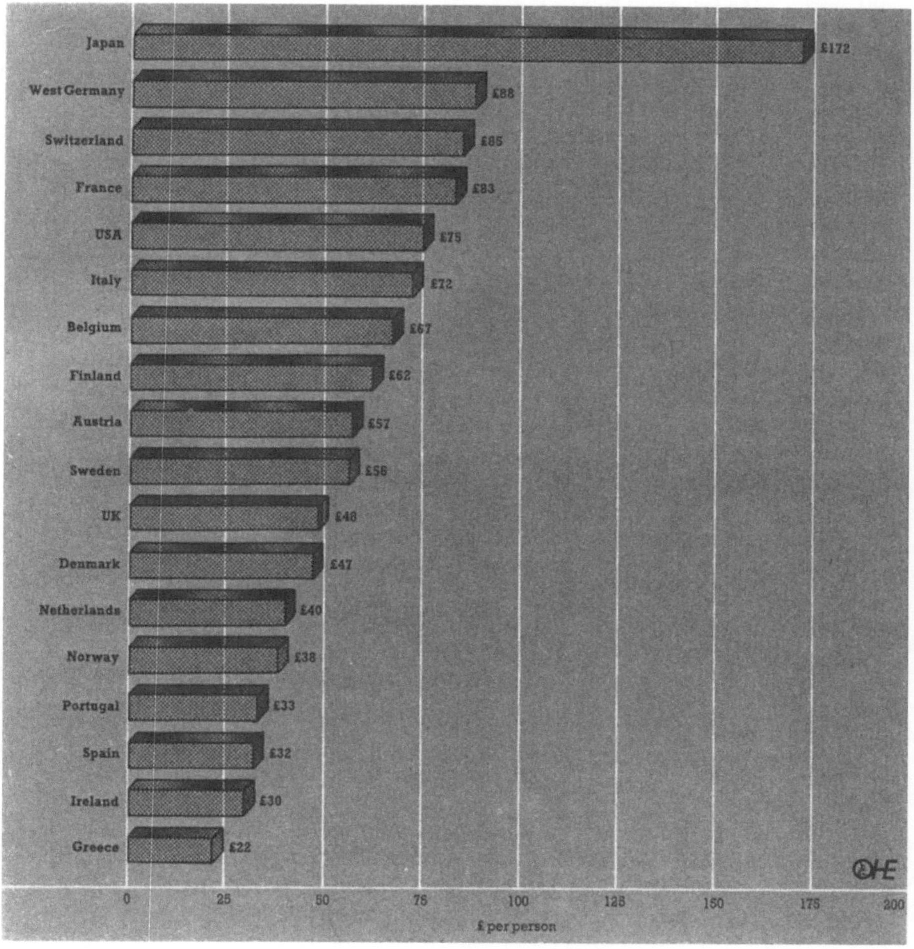

Note: All figures include prescription sales (plus hospital) as well as over-the-counter medicines, and consumption figures may be affected by foreign exchange fluctuations.

Sources: EFPIA, PMA, and JPMA.

From Compendium of Health Statistics, 7th Edition, 1989. Published by the Office of Health Economics, London. Reproduced by kind permission of the Director.

INDEX

MIX
Papier aus verantwortungsvollen Quellen
Paper from responsible sources
FSC® C105338

If you have any concerns about our products,
you can contact us on
ProductSafety@springernature.com

In case Publisher is established outside the EU,
the EU authorized representative is:
Springer Nature Customer Service Center GmbH
Europaplatz 3, 69115 Heidelberg, Germany

Printed by Libri Plureos GmbH
in Hamburg, Germany